Breast Imaging Cases

below

Published and Forthcoming books in the
Cases in Radiology **series:**

Breast Imaging Cases

Catherine M. Appleton, MD

Assistant Professor, Radiology
Mallinckrodt Institute of Radiology
Washington University School of Medicine
St. Louis, Missouri

Kimberly N. Wiele, MD

Assistant Professor, Radiology
Mallinckrodt Institute of Radiology
Washington University School of Medicine
St. Louis, Missouri

With contributions from
Susan Holley, MD, PhD

Clinical Instructor
Mallinckrodt Institute of Radiology
Washington University School of Medicine
St. Louis, Missouri

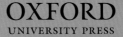

OXFORD
UNIVERSITY PRESS

OXFORD
UNIVERSITY PRESS

Oxford University Press, Inc., publishes works that further
Oxford University's objective of excellence
in research, scholarship, and education.

Oxford   New York
Auckland   Cape Town   Dar es Salaam   Hong Kong   Karachi
Kuala Lumpur   Madrid   Melbourne   Mexico City   Nairobi
New Delhi   Shanghai   Taipei   Toronto

With offices in
Argentina   Austria   Brazil   Chile   Czech Republic   France   Greece
Guatemala   Hungary   Italy   Japan   Poland   Portugal   Singapore
South Korea   Switzerland   Thailand   Turkey   Ukraine   Vietnam

Copyright © 2012 by Oxford University Press, Inc.

Published by Oxford University Press, Inc.
198 Madison Avenue, New York, New York 10016
www.oup.com

Oxford is a registered trademark of Oxford University Press

Library of Congress Cataloging-in-Publication Data

Appleton, Catherine M.
Breast imaging cases / Catherine M. Appleton, Kimberly N. Wiele ;
with image contributions from Susan Holley.
p. ; cm. — (Cases in radiology)
Includes bibliographical references and index.
ISBN 978-0-19-973192-3
1. Breast—Imaging—Case studies. 2. Breast—Diseases—Diagnosis—Case studies.
I. Wiele, Kimberly N. II. Title. III. Series: Cases in radiology.
[DNLM: 1. Breast Diseases—diagnosis—Case Reports. 2. Breast Neoplasms—diagnosis—Case Reports.
3. Diagnostic Imaging—Case Reports. WP 815]
RG493.5.D52A67   2011
618.1'90757—dc22
2011012637

9 8 7 6 5 4 3 2 1
Printed in China
on acid-free paper

For my parents, who always told me I could do anything; my husband, who champions my efforts, and my children, Lily and Mack, who make it all worthwhile. **CMA**

To my biggest fan and husband, Bob, and my 3 incredible children, Ben, Greg and Amanda. **KNW**

For my teachers, with gratitude; for my family, with love. **SH**

Contents

Preface

This book provides a case-based, high yield, easy-to-read format presenting a spectrum of breast pathology presented through multiple imaging modalities. Generally, the cases are presented in order of increasing difficulty, although the respective difficulty may be relative to each reader. This text is certainly not intended to be comprehensive; however, classic and common diagnoses that a general practice radiologist would expect to encounter are featured. A few uncommon or rare cases are included for interest. The final 10 cases are dedicated to breast MR. They are grouped in order to have over-lapping and inclusive teaching points. We hope this book will serve in preparation for breast-imaging rotations, exams and the practice of radiology.

Acknowledgments

We gratefully acknowledge Barbara Monsees, MD, for building and developing the Breast Health Center at Barnes-Jewish Hospital/Washington University School of Medicine in St. Louis. She fosters a work environment encouraging world-class breast imaging each and every day. She supports us in our professional pursuits and remains a woman we each call friend.

We also thank Mary Kay Stemmler, RT(R)(M) for her assistance in obtaining many of the images contained in this volume.

The Publisher thanks the following for their time and advice:

Mark Anderson, University of Virginia

Sanjeev Bhalla, Mallinckrodt Institute of Radiology, Washington University

Michael Bruno, Penn State Hershey Medical Center

Melissa Rosado de Christenson, St. Luke's Hospital of Kansas City

Rihan Khan, University of Arizona

Angela Levy, Georgetown University

Alexander Mamourian, University of Pennsylvania

Stacy Smith, Brigham and Women's Hospital

History

► Screening mammogram

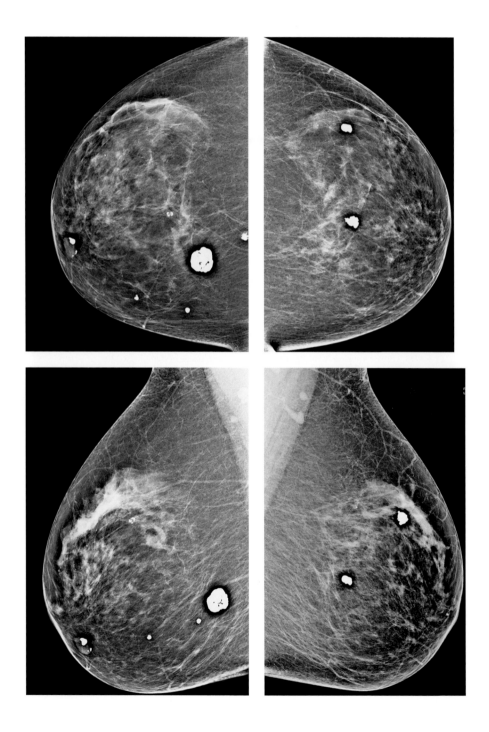

Case 1 Benign Calcifications from Involuting Fibroadenomas

Findings

► Bilateral coarse or "popcorn" calcifications

Differential Diagnosis

► None—classic appearance for involuting/hyalinizing fibroadenomas demonstrated

Teaching Points

► Hyalinizing fibroademonas frequently demonstrate a decrease in size of the circumscribed mass, with the associated development of dense, coarse, "popcorn" calcifications
► Calcifications are typically large (>3 mm), dense, and coarse
► Frequently multiple and bilateral but can occur in isolation
► May have residual associated soft tissue density or mass

Management

► BI-RADS® Category 2: Benign finding
► Annual screening mammography

Selected References/Further Reading

Bassett LW, et al. *Diagnosis of Diseases of the Breast*, 2nd ed. Philadelphia: WB Saunders, 2005:424-428.

Cardenosa G. *Clinical Breast Imaging: A Patient-Focused Teaching File*. Philadelphia: Lippincott Williams & Wilkins, 2007:19-22.

D'Orsi CJ, Bassett LW, Berg WA, et al. BI-RADS: Mammography, 4th edition in: D'Orsi CJ, Mendelson EB, Ikeda DM, et al: Breast Imaging Reporting and Data System: ACR BI-RADS – Breast Imaging Atlas, Reston, VA, American College of Radiology, 2003.

History

► 50-year-old woman with a palpable mass in the left breast, 10 o'clock position

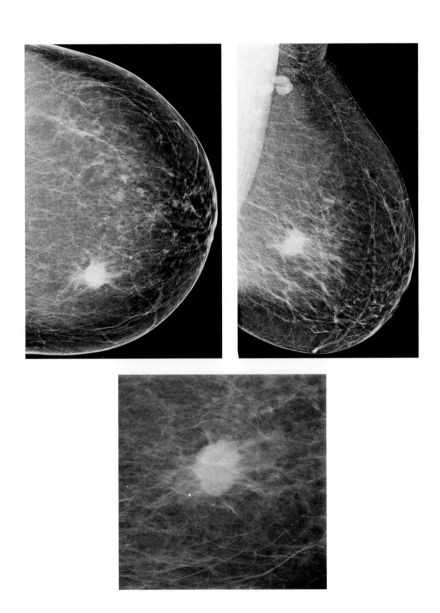

Case 2 Invasive Ductal Carcinoma with Metastatic Axillary Lymph Node

Findings

► There is a dense, lobular mass with indistinct margins and associated amorphous microcalcifications in the left breast, 10 o'clock position (correlating to the palpable area of concern)
► There is an enlarged axillary lymph node with thickened cortex

Differential Diagnosis

► Papillary carcinoma
► Given the presence of microcalcifications, invasive lobular carcinoma is less likely (microcalcifications are not a typical feature of lobular carcinoma)

Teaching Points

► Magnification views are helpful to delineate extent of disease (particularly when there are microcalcifications associated with a suspicious mass)
► Ultrasound of the mass (not shown in this case) should be performed to allow planning for percutaneous core needle biopsy
► Ultrasound of the ipsilateral axilla should be performed for all highly suspicious breast masses
  ▪ Can detect non-palpable abnormal lymph nodes
► Once the diagnosis is confirmed, contrast-enhanced MR should be considered to further evaluate extent of disease in the affected breast, and for ancillary screening of the contralateral breast

Management

► BI-RADS® Category 5: Highly suspicious for malignancy
► Ultrasound-guided core needle biopsy of the mass and fine-needle aspiration (FNA) of the suspicious axillary lymph node
  ▪ If the lymph node FNA yields metastatic disease, then sentinel lymph node sampling is not performed; the patient would undergo axillary lymph node dissection

Selected References/Further Reading

Bassett LW, et al. *Diagnosis of Diseases of the Breast*, 2nd ed. Philadelphia: WB Saunders Co., 2005:485-490.
Ikeda DM. *Breast Imaging: The Requisites*. Philadelphia: Elsevier Mosby, 2004:116-117.
Stavros AT. *Breast Ultrasound*. Philadelphia: Lippincott Williams & Wilkins, 2004:838-847.

History

▶ Screening mammogram

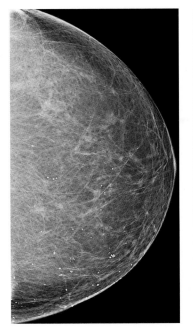 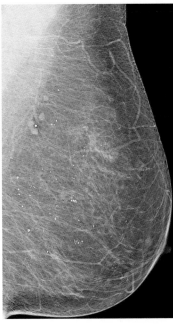

Case 3 Dermal Calcifications

Findings

► Diffusely scattered, benign, skin calcifications

Differential Diagnosis

► None—classic appearance demonstrated

Teaching Points

► Dermal calcifications are typically lucent-centered or "eggshell" in appearance, polygonal in shape, 1 to 2 mm in size
► Arise from dermal sweat glands
► Most commonly found in the axilla, medial breast, or inframammary fold
► Classic findings need not be described in screening exam reports
  ▪ If you are uncertain that clustered microcalcifications are dermal in location, magnification tangential views should be performed
  ▪ If calcifications are confirmed to be within the skin, no further workup is required

Management

► Annual screening mammography

Selected References/Further Reading

Bassett LW, et al. *Diagnosis of Diseases of the Breast*, 2nd ed. Philadelphia: WB Saunders Co., 2005:402-405.

Ikeda DM. *Breast Imaging: The Requisites*. Philadelphia: Elsevier Mosby, 2004:73-75.

D'Orsi CJ, Bassett LW, Berg WA, et al. BI-RADS: Mammography, 4th edition in: D'Orsi CJ, Mendelson EB, Ikeda DM, et al: Breast Imaging Reporting and Data System: ACR BI-RADS – Breast Imaging Atlas, Reston, VA, American College of Radiology, 2003.

History

▶ Screening mammogram (right breast images shown)

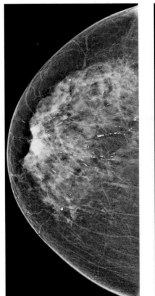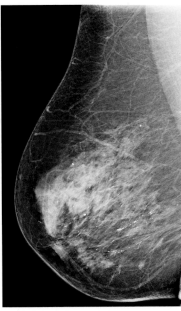

Case 4 Secretory Calcifications

Findings

► Extensive, dense, "rod-like" calcifications in ductal distributions. Note the nipple retraction (long-standing per the patient's history)

Differential Diagnosis

► Classic appearance demonstrated

Teaching Points

► Benign
  ▪ Usually women >60 years
► Classically solid or discontinuous smooth, linear, rod-like calcifications
  ▪ Deposited in distended debris-filled ducts
  ▪ Usually bilateral and symmetric
  ▪ May appear lucent-centered
  ▪ Ductal distribution towards the nipple
► Also known as plasma cell mastitis
► May have associated nipple retraction
► Asymptomatic and inconsequential
  ▪ Occasionally, diagnostic evaluation with magnification views is needed to further define morphology and exclude "casting" ductal carcinoma in situ (DCIS)
    ◆ When scant, unilateral, or with atypical features
► *Rarely,* atypical appearance may warrant stereotactic core needle biopsy to exclude DCIS

Management

► BI-RADS® Category 2: Benign finding
► Annual screening mammography

Selected References/Further Reading

Bassett LW, et al. *Diagnosis of Diseases of the Breast*, 2nd ed. Philadelphia: WB Saunders Co., 2005:443-445 and 484.

Sickles EA. Breast calcifications: mammographic evaluation. *Radiology* 1986;160:289-293.

D'Orsi CJ, Bassett LW, Berg WA, et al. BI-RADS: Mammography, 4th edition in: D'Orsi CJ, Mendelson EB, Ikeda DM, et al: Breast Imaging Reporting and Data System: ACR BI-RADS – Breast Imaging Atlas, Reston, VA, American College of Radiology, 2003.

History

▶ 48-year-old woman with a tender palpable mass in the right breast, upper outer quadrant

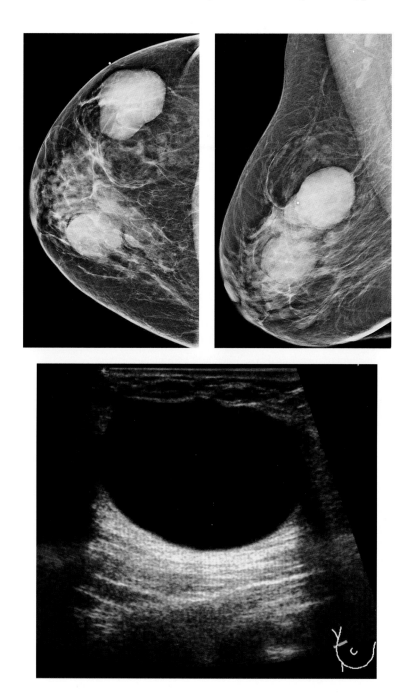

Case 5   Simple Cyst

Findings

- ► Mammogram: The palpable mass is marked with a metallic BB and corresponds with a circumscribed, oval equal-density mass. There is a second (similar-appearing) mass noted incidentally in the upper inner quadrant
- ► Ultrasound: The palpable mass corresponds with a circumscribed, anechoic, oval, parallel mass with imperceptible wall and marked posterior acoustic enhancement

Differential Diagnosis

- ► None—classic appearance demonstrated given ultrasound findings

Teaching Points

- ► Most common breast mass; often multiple and bilateral but can occur in isolation
- ► Circumscribed, low- or equal-density, round or oval masses on mammogram
    - ▪ May have obscured margins in dense glandular tissue
- ► Ultrasound is the definitive imaging tool to confirm a simple cyst
    - ▪ Mammography cannot distinguish cysts from solid circumscribed masses
- ► *Simple* cysts are benign
    - ▪ Must be *anechoic* to characterize as a simple cyst
    - ▪ Aspiration of simple cysts can be performed when painful, for symptomatic relief
- ► *Complicated* cysts have similar ultrasound features but contain low-level internal echoes
    - ▪ Consider aspiration of *complicated* cysts when new, painful, or enlarging

Management

- ► BI-RADS® Category 2: Benign finding
- ► Reassure patient
- ► Annual screening mammography

Selected References/Further Reading

Bassett LW, et al. *Diagnosis of Diseases of the Breast*, 2nd ed. Philadelphia: WB Saunders Co., 2005:433-437.

Ikeda DM. *Breast Imaging: The Requisites*. Philadelphia: Elsevier Mosby, 2004:122-124.

Stavros AT. *Breast Ultrasound*. Philadelphia: Lippincott Williams & Wilkins, 2004; Chapter 10.

History

▶ 46-year-old male with a tender, left breast mass

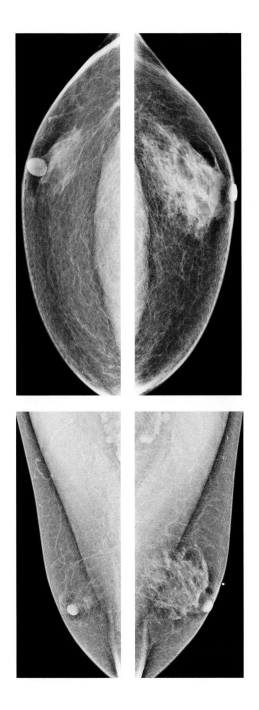

Case 6 Gynecomastia

Findings

▶ A metallic BB denotes the area of palpable concern in the left breast. There is asymmetric "flame-shaped" density, in the left subareolar breast consistent with glandular tissue. (There is minimal glandular tissue in the right subareolar breast, which went unnoticed by the patient.)

Differential Diagnosis

▶ None—classic appearance of benign gynecomastia demonstrated
▶ In male patients, may consider
  ▪ Male breast cancer: typically presents as a mass, frequently with spiculated margins (similar appearance to invasive breast cancer in female patients)
    ◆ Far less common than gynecomastia
  ▪ Pseudogynecomastia: fatty enlargement secondary to obesity
    ◆ Fat density mammographically

Teaching Points

▶ Gynecomastia is the proliferation of ductal and stromal elements resulting in breast enlargement in males
▶ Common causes include systemic disease (e.g., liver disease, HIV infection) and side effects from drugs (e.g., digitalis, spironolactone, marijuana, anabolic steroids)
  ▪ Frequently idiopathic and may spontaneously regress
  ▪ If the precipitating cause is corrected, may be reversible in early stages
▶ Clinical exam and correlation with risk factors may prove helpful
▶ Common finding on clinical exam
  ▪ Accounts for 85% of masses in male patients
▶ May occur at any age (tri-modal distribution described when hormonal in origin)
  ▪ Neonate (maternal estrogen stimulation)
  ▪ Pubertal (estradiol surge)
  ▪ Older men (decreasing testosterone)
▶ Mammographic patterns include nodular, dendritic, and diffuse glandular
▶ Ultrasound has a less specific appearance (hypoechoic subareolar tissue)
▶ If the precipitating cause is corrected, may be reversible in early stages

Management

▶ Clinical follow-up, with evaluation of any underlying condition that could precipitate gynecomastia. No further imaging is required

Selected References/Further Reading

Bassett LW, et al. *Diagnosis of Diseases of the Breast*, 2nd ed. Philadelphia: WB Saunders Co., 2005:539-549.
Cardenosa G. *Clinical Breast Imaging: A Patient-Focused Teaching File*. Philadelphia: Lippincott Williams & Wilkins, 2007:308-309.
Ikeda DM. *Breast Imaging: The Requisites*. Philadelphia: Elsevier Mosby, 2004:279-284.

History

▶ 46-year-old woman with a palpable mass in the right breast (a metallic BB marks the area of concern)

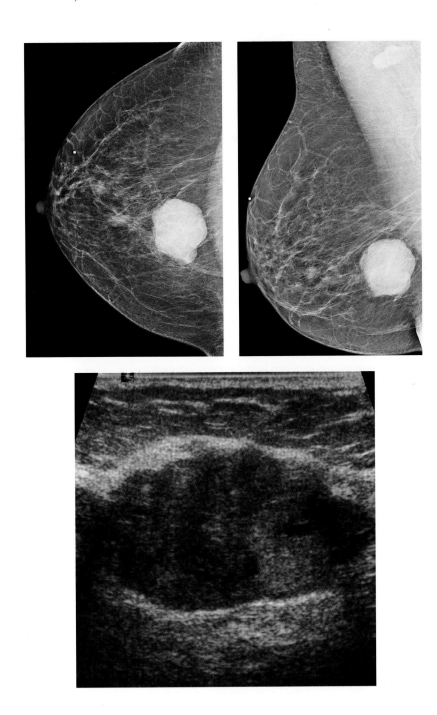

Case 7 Invasive Mucinous (Colloid) Carcinoma

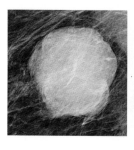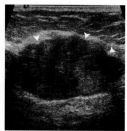

Findings

- ▶ Mammogram: Large, high-density, lobular, circumscribed mass in the deep central breast
- ▶ Ultrasound: Heterogeneous predominantly hypoechoic mass with microlobulated borders (*arrowheads*) and associated posterior acoustic enhancement

Differential Diagnosis

- ▶ Phyllodes tumor
- ▶ Fibroadenoma
- ▶ Medullary cancer

Teaching Points

- ▶ Favorable prognosis
- ▶ Accounts for <5% of breast cancers, more common in older women
- ▶ May appear low density, or iso-dense to surrounding glandular tissue
- ▶ Typically a slow-growing, round, circumscribed mass
  - ▪ Magnification mammography may reveal an indistinct margin
- ▶ May mimic a complicated or complex cyst at ultrasound
  - ▪ Careful attention to all margins during ultrasound is crucial to avoid misdiagnosis
- ▶ Although posterior acoustic enhancement is a typical characteristic of cystic masses, it may also be a feature of certain *solid* breast masses including high-grade invasive ductal carcinoma and mucinous carcinoma
- ▶ Although breast malignancies often demonstrate irregular or spiculated margins, some will present with circumscribed margins including:
  - ▪ High-grade invasive ductal carcinoma
  - ▪ Mucinous carcinoma
  - ▪ Phyllodes tumor
  - ▪ Primary breast lymphoma
  - ▪ Metastasis

Management

- ▶ Ultrasound-guided core needle biopsy is recommended for diagnosis

Selected References/Further Reading

Bassett LW, et al. *Diagnosis of Diseases of the Breast*, 2nd ed. Philadelphia: WB Saunders Co., 2005:504-506.
Ikeda DM. *Breast Imaging: The Requisites*. Philadelphia: Elsevier Mosby, 2004:145-147.
Stavros AT. *Breast Ultrasound*. Philadelphia: Lippincott Williams & Wilkins, 2004:645-648.

History

▶ Annual diagnostic mammogram in a patient with a history of breast conservation therapy (BCT)

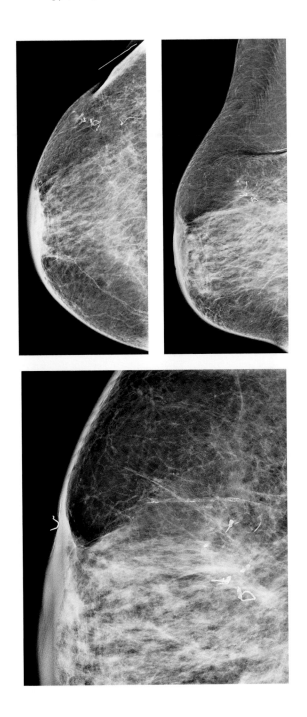

Case 8 Suture Calcifications

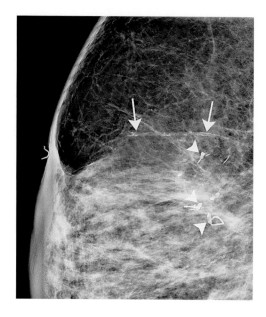

Findings

▶ Ring-like, curvilinear and linear calcified suture material in the previous lumpectomy site (note the calcified knots, *arrowheads*)

▶ Vascular calcifications are noted incidentally (*arrows*)

Differential Diagnosis

▶ None—classic appearance demonstrated

Teaching Points

▶ Uncommon

▶ May see calcified knots, which confirms the diagnosis

▶ Most commonly seen in patients following lumpectomy and radiation therapy

▶ May occur after reduction mammoplasty

Management

▶ BI-RADS® Category 2: Benign finding

▶ Annual diagnostic mammography (given history of breast conservation therapy)

Further Reading/Selected References

Bassett LW, et al. *Diagnosis of Diseases of the Breast*, 2nd ed. Philadelphia: WB Saunders Co., 2005:618.

Ikeda DM. *Breast Imaging: The Requisites*. Philadelphia: Elsevier Mosby, 2004:314-315.

Kopans DB. *Atlas of Breast Imaging*. Philadelphia: Lippincott Williams & Wilkins, 1999:33.

History

▶ 47-year-old woman with a palpable mass in the left breast, upper inner quadrant

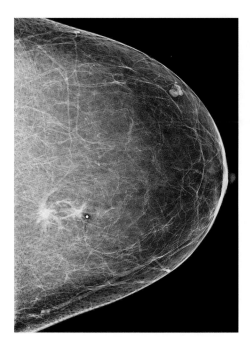
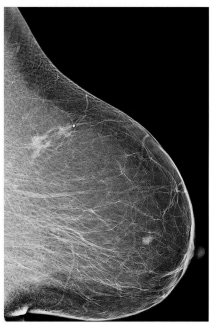

Case 9 Invasive Ductal Carcinoma with Ductal Carcinoma In Situ (DCIS)

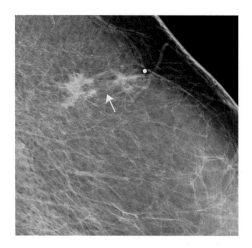

Findings

▶ There are two adjacent, irregular masses with spiculated margins and associated intervening linear calcifications (*arrow*)

Differential Diagnosis

▶ Classic appearance of invasive ductal carcinoma with DCIS demonstrated

Teaching Points

▶ Invasive ductal cancer is classically an irregular mass with spiculated margins
 ▪ May be new or enlarging
▶ Invasive ductal cancers frequently have associated microcalcifications
 ▪ Calcifications usually represent the intraductal portion (DCIS)
 ▪ Magnified images should be performed to delineate full extent of microcalcifications
  ◆ Crucial for surgical planning
▶ IDC can present as a palpable mass, or be detected on screening mammogram
▶ "Multi-focal" breast cancer is used to describe two or more foci of cancer in the same quadrant

Management

▶ BI-RADS® Category 5: Highly suspicious for malignancy
▶ Ultrasound-guided or stereotactic-guided core biopsy prior to definitive surgical treatment
▶ Given the extent of disease, a two-needle bracket localization is recommended to reduce the risk of positive surgical margins

Selected References/Further Reading

Bassett LW, et al. *Diagnosis of Diseases of the Breast,* 2nd ed. Philadelphia: WB Saunders Co., 2005:485-499, 509.
Ikeda DM. *Breast Imaging: The Requisites*. Philadelphia: Elsevier Mosby, 2004:81-84.

History

► Previous right breast conservation therapy (BCT). Annual diagnostic mammogram

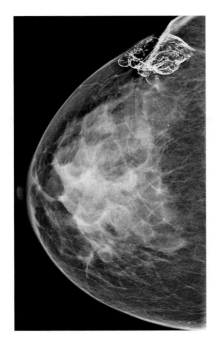 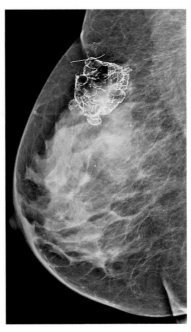

Case 10 Fat Necrosis after Breast Conservation Therapy

Findings

▶ In the upper outer quadrant, there is a large lobular mass containing fat centrally with associated peripheral rim calcification

Differential Diagnosis

▶ Classic appearance demonstrated
  ▪ However, early calcification of fat necrosis may mimic microcalcifications of malignancy

Teaching Points

▶ Varied mammographic appearance
  ▪ Most commonly presents as a radiolucent or mixed-density (fat and soft tissue) circumscribed mass with associated rim calcifications ("oil cyst")
  ▪ Mimics lipoma when non-calcified
▶ Evolving fat necrosis in the operative site is common
▶ Commonly occurs after trauma or surgery (breast conserving surgery, reduction mammoplasty)
  ▪ But may occur without any history of surgery or trauma
▶ May be detected incidentally, or present as a palpable mass
  ▪ Clinical findings may be suspicious (firm, palpable mass)
▶ Occasionally appears as architectural distortion or mass-like
  ▪ Atypical imaging features may warrant diagnostic evaluation and possible biopsy

Management

▶ Ultrasound often confusing and not helpful in most cases
▶ With classic appearance biopsy can be avoided

Selected References/Further Reading

Bassett LW, et al. *Diagnosis of Diseases of the Breast*, 2nd ed. Philadelphia: WB Saunders Co., 2005:409-419.
Cardenosa G. *Clinical Breast Imaging: A Patient-Focused Teaching File*. Philadelphia: Lippincott Williams & Wilkins, 2007:371-373.
Ikeda DM. *Breast Imaging: The Requisites*. Philadelphia: Elsevier Mosby, 2004:100-1034.

History

▶ Screening mammogram

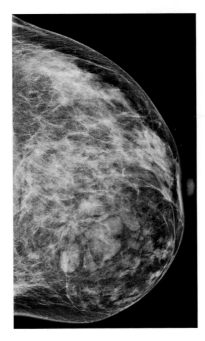 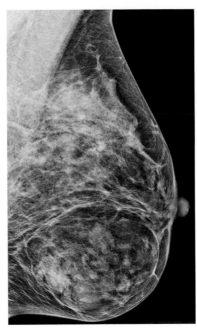

Case 11   Fibroadenolipoma (Hamartoma)

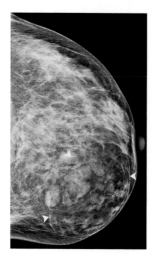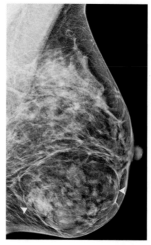

Findings

▸ There is a large encapsulated mass in the lower inner quadrant (*arrowheads*) containing both fat and glandular elements ("breast within a breast" or "cut-sausage" appearance)

Differential Diagnosis

▸ None—classic appearance demonstrated

Teaching Points

▸ Typically incidental finding, but rarely presents as a palpable mass
▸ When sparse fat components are present, fibroadenoma may be suspected
▸ "Don't touch" lesion when classic features are present
▸ Ultrasound rarely required but can demonstrate heterogeneous glandular and fat components, with a thin echogenic pseudocapsule
▸ Other common fat-containing breast masses include:
  ▪ Lipoma
  ▪ Galactocele
  ▪ Intramammary lymph node
  ▪ Oil cyst

Management

▸ BI-RADS® Category 2: Benign finding
▸ Annual screening mammography

Selected References/Further Reading

American College of Radiology (ACR). ACR BI-RADS®—Mammography, 4th ed. *ACR Breast Imaging Reporting and Data Systems, Breast Imaging Atlas.* Reston, VA. American College of Radiology, 2003:62-65.

Bassett LW, et al. *Diagnosis of Diseases of the Breast*, 2nd ed. Philadelphia: WB Saunders Co., 2005:430-432.

Stavros AT. *Breast Ultrasound*. Philadelphia: Lippincott Williams & Wilkins, 2004:560-569.

History

► 46-year-old asymptomatic woman undergoing annual screening mammogram

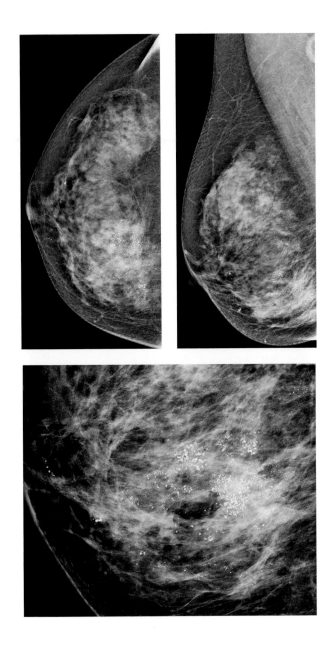

Case 12   High-grade (Grade 3/3) Ductal Carcinoma In Situ (DCIS)

Findings

- ▶ There are pleomorphic microcalcifications in a segmental distribution involving most of the right lower inner quadrant (greater than 5 cm)
- ▶ There is associated soft tissue density in the lower inner quadrant, some of which appears tubular (ductal) in appearance

Differential Diagnosis

- ▶ None—classic appearance demonstrated (the microcalcifications represent the ductal carcinoma growing within the ducts)

Teaching Points

- ▶ DCIS is usually detected on screening mammography
  - ▪ Rarely can present as a palpable mass
- ▶ Stage 0 (non-invasive) cancer
  - ▪ Staging is determined at the time of definitive surgery
  - ▪ Even if core biopsy reveals only DCIS, lumpectomy or mastectomy may reveal an invasive component of malignancy
- ▶ Segmentally distributed calcifications should be regarded with suspicion,
  - ▪ May be benign or malignant
  - ▪ Careful analysis of morphology is required
- ▶ Suspicious microcalcifications can be sampled using stereotactic vacuum-assisted core needle biopsy
  - ▪ When there is associated soft tissue density, or calcifications extend more than 25 mm, consider ultrasound to survey for an underlying mass (which may represent an underlying invasive component)

Management

- ▶ Stereotactic biopsy is recommended to establish diagnosis
- ▶ Given the extent of disease in this patient, mastectomy for definitive surgical treatment is recommended (however, most patients with less extensive DCIS will be candidates for breast conservation therapy)

Selected References/Further Reading

American College of Radiology (ACR). ACR BI-RADS®—Mammography, 4th ed. *ACR Breast Imaging Reporting and Data Systems, Breast Imaging Atlas*. Reston, VA. American College of Radiology, 2003:124-127.

Ikeda DM. *Breast Imaging: The Requisites*. Philadelphia: Elsevier Mosby, 2004:60-70.

Tabar L, et al. *Breast Cancer: The Art and Science of Early Detection with Mammography*. New York: Thieme, 2005:106-108.

History

▶ Screening mammogram (cropped images shown)

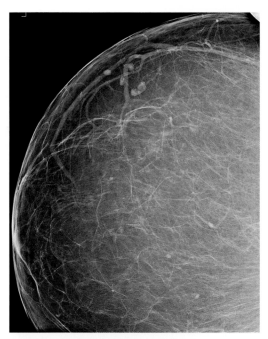

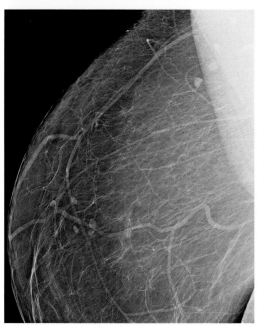

Case 13 Benign Intramammary Lymph Nodes

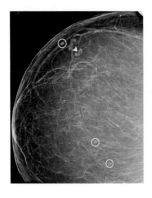 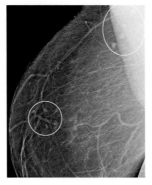

Findings

► Multiple reniform circumscribed fat-containing masses (*small circles*) in the right breast parenchyma and axilla (*large circle*)
► Note the fatty hilum (*arrowhead*)

Differential Diagnosis

► Classic appearance demonstrated
► If fatty hilum cannot be seen, may mimic solid benign or malignant mass

Teaching Points

► Very common; typically occur in the lateral portion of the upper outer quadrant
► Usually incidental, but can present as palpable mass
► Frequently multiple
► Usually less than a centimeter, but can be larger
► Classic appearance mammographically
  ▪ Viewed tangentially, reniform shape with a fatty hilum
  ▪ Viewed *en face*, fatty hilum will be central
► If classic appearance is not demonstrated mammographically, ultrasound may be helpful
  ▪ Ultrasound appearance: oval, circumscribed, parallel mass with hypoechoic cortex, echogenic hilum and feeding vessel
► Contrast-enhanced MR will routinely demonstrate "washout" enhancement kinetics
  ▪ To avoid mistaking for a suspicious finding, correlate with the fat-suppressed image to identify the classic reniform shape and central fatty hilum

Management

► Classic appearance requires no further evaluation
► Annual screening mammography

Selected References/Further Reading

Bassett LW, et al. *Diagnosis of Diseases of the Breast*, 2nd ed. Philadelphia: WB Saunders Co., 2005:407-409.
Kopans DB. *Atlas of Breast Imaging*. Philadelphia: Lippincott Williams & Wilkins, 1999:64-65, 124-125.
Morris EA, Liberman L. *Breast MRI: Diagnosis and Intervention*. New York: Springer, 2005:123.
Stavros AT. *Breast Ultrasound*. Philadelphia: Lippincott Williams & Wilkins, 2004:847-853.

History

► Screening mammogram

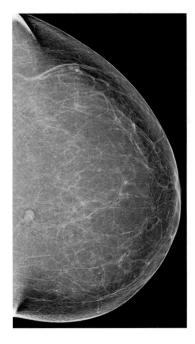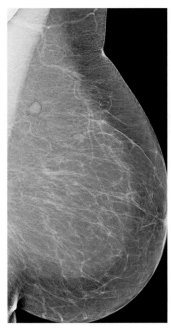

Case 14 Skin Lesion

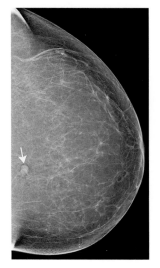 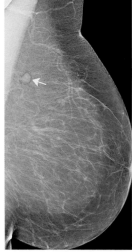 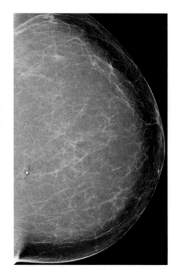

Findings

► Standard images demonstrate a circumscribed, iso-dense, round mass in the upper central breast with a surrounding lucent halo or "air crescent" (*arrow*)
► A metallic BB was placed on a raised nevus to demonstrate that the "mass" is actually a raised skin lesion

Differential Diagnosis

► True mass within the breast parenchyma

Teaching Points

► Skin lesions can project over the breast and appear to represent intraparenchymal masses
► Technologists should diagram raised skin lesions or affix lesions with radiopaque markers (unless numerous lesions are present, such as a patient with neurofibromatosis)
► Some lesions (seborrheic keratosis) may contain reticulated lucencies or hyperdense debris and are less likely to be mistaken for a parenchymal mass
► Keloid scars can occur following breast surgery
  ▪ Appear as raised tubular masses along incision lines

Management

► After confirmation of a skin lesion (either with physical exam or with placement of a radiopaque marker) no additional evaluation is warranted
► Annual screening mammography

Selected References/Further Reading

Bassett LW, et al. *Diagnosis of Diseases of the Breast*, 2nd ed. Philadelphia: WB Saunders Co., 2005:399-401.
Cardenosa G. *Clinical Breast Imaging: A Patient-Focused Teaching File*. Philadelphia: Lippincott Williams & Wilkins, 2007:2-5.
Ikeda DM. *Breast Imaging: The Requisites*. Philadelphia: Elsevier Mosby, 2004:70-71.

History

▸ Post-excision mammogram following lumpectomy for invasive ductal carcinoma (IDC)

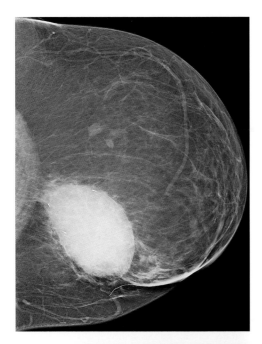

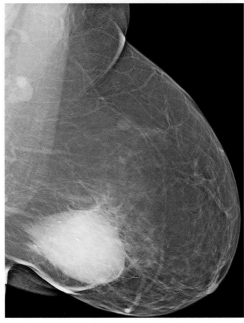

Case 15 Seroma Following Lumpectomy

Findings

- There is an oval, circumscribed, high-density mass in the upper inner quadrant at the lumpectomy site (a linear metallic scar marker is present)
- Multiple surgical clips are present at the edges of the mass

Differential Diagnosis

- Hematoma

Teaching Points

- Seroma and hematoma occur commonly following excisional biopsy/lumpectomy
- Seroma is an accumulation of serous fluid in the biopsy cavity
  - If rapidly enlarging, surgical evacuation may be required to exclude active hemorrhage/hematoma
- Air–fluid levels can be seen in the acute postoperative period
- Typically self-limited and diminish in size and mammographic density over time
  - Growth or increased density should be regarded with suspicion
- Ultrasound usually demonstrates a fluid collection with debris and thin movable septa
- Breast conservation therapy (BCT) describes surgical removal of a malignancy (lumpectomy) and subsequent radiation treatment
  - Broad spectrum of mammographic findings after BCT, including architectural distortion, stromal/trabecular thickening, fat necrosis, skin thickening, global increased density (and decreased compressibility)
  - Conspicuity of findings usually decreases over several years but can be chronic

Management

- Aspiration of postoperative seroma can usually be avoided but may be performed if the patient is symptomatic
- Radiation therapy and subsequent annual diagnostic mammography

Selected References/Further Reading

Bassett LW, et al. *Diagnosis of Diseases of the Breast*, 2nd ed. Philadelphia: WB Saunders Co., 2005:570-571.

Bland K, Copeland E. *The Breast: Comprehensive Management of Benign and Malignant Disorders*, 3rd ed. Philadelphia: WB Saunders Co., 2004:957-958.

Ikeda DM. *Breast Imaging: The Requisites*. Philadelphia: Elsevier Mosby, 2004:239-2464.

History

► Palpable mass in the right superior central breast (indicated by a metallic BB)

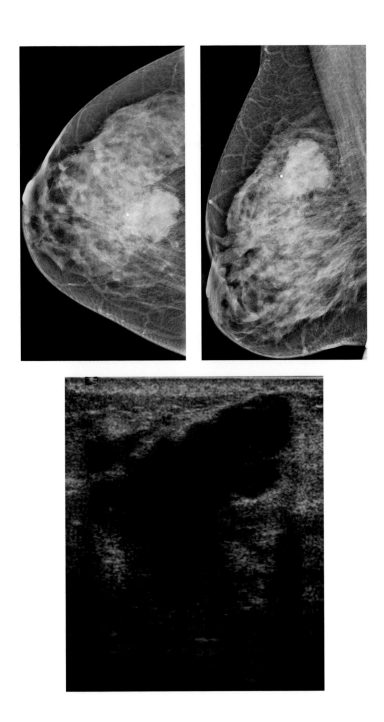

Case 16 Invasive Lobular Carcinoma (ILC)

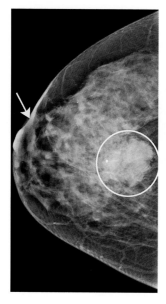
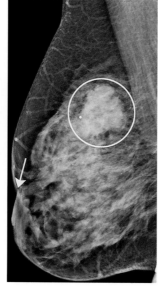

Findings

▶ Mammogram: Metallic BB marks a high-density lobular mass with partially circumscribed, partially obscured margins in the upper central right breast (*circles*)
  - The patient is status post remote benign excisional biopsy resulting in skin thickening and distortion anteriorly (*arrows*)
▶ Ultrasound: Irregular, hypoechoic solid mass with microlobulated margins with a non-parallel orientation

Differential Diagnosis

▶ Invasive ductal carcinoma
▶ Medullary carcinoma
▶ Phyllodes tumor
▶ Atypical presentation of fibroadenoma (much less likely)

Teaching Points

▶ May present as palpable mass or "thickening"
▶ Accounts for less than 10% of all invasive breast cancers
▶ Higher rate of multifocal, multicentric, and/or bilateral involvement compared to invasive ductal cancer (IDC)
▶ ILC has a variable appearance mammographically
  - Iso-dense or high-density mass with spiculated or indistinct margins
  - Architectural distortion
  - Developing density
  - Can be a one-view finding
  - Microcalcifications NOT a characteristic feature

- Variable appearance on ultrasound
  - Hypoechoic irregular mass (shown in this case)
  - Diffuse acoustic shadowing
    - More common with larger tumors
- Tumor cells grow in single-file lines, infiltrating between collagen bundles
  - This growth pattern is thought to contribute to the subtle presentation of some tumors
  - Notoriously difficult to detect mammographically

Management

- BI-RADS® Category 5: Highly suspicious for malignancy
- Ultrasound-guided core-needle biopsy for tissue diagnosis
- When diagnosis of ILC is confirmed, contrast-enhanced MR should be considered
  - Delineate extent of disease for surgical planning
  - Evaluate the contralateral breast for clinically and mammographically occult disease

Selected References/Further Reading

Bassett LW, et al. *Diagnosis of Diseases of the Breast*, 2nd ed. Philadelphia: WB Saunders Co., 2005:499-500.
Ikeda DM. *Breast Imaging: The Requisites.* Philadelphia: Elsevier Mosby, 2004:97-98.
Tabar L et al. *Breast Cancer: The Art and Science of Early Detection with Mammography.*
   New York: Thieme, 2005:372-377.

History

▶ Screening mammogram

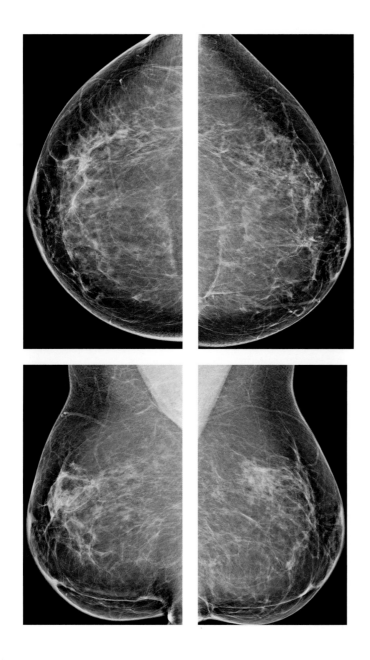

Case 17 Reduction Mammoplasty (Breast Reduction)

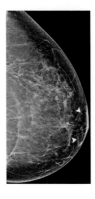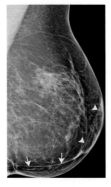

Findings

▸ Note the subareolar fibrotic band (*arrowheads*), elevation of the nipple, "swirling" of the glandular tissue due to surgical relocation (*arrows*), and paucity of breast tissue in the lower breast

Differential Diagnosis

▸ None—classic findings are demonstrated

Teaching Points

▸ Elective plastic surgery procedure
  ▪ To treat macromastia
  ▪ To achieve symmetry in patients following contralateral breast cancer surgery (breast conservation therapy or mastectomy with reconstruction)
  ▪ To address congenital asymmetry
▸ Variable techniques described
  ▪ Circumareolar ("keyhole") incision most commonly employed
▸ Overall breast density may be reduced when compared with pre-reduction exams
▸ Other classic imaging findings (not seen in this case) include
  ▪ Fat necrosis with dystrophic calcifications and oil cysts
  ▪ Skin calcifications along suture lines
  ▪ Architectural distortion
  ▪ Skin thickening
  ▪ Altered breast contour
▸ Preoperative mammogram recommended to exclude occult malignancy
▸ Mammaplasty and mammoplasty are both accepted spelling

Management

▸ BI-RADS® Category 2: Benign findings
▸ Annual screening mammography

Selected References/Further Reading

Bassett LW, et al. *Diagnosis of Diseases of the Breast*, 2nd ed. Philadelphia: WB Saunders Co., 2005: Chapter 33.

Bland K, Copeland E. *The Breast: Comprehensive Management of Benign and Malignant Disorders*, 3rd ed. Philadelphia: WB Saunders Co., 2004: Chapter 44.

Ikeda DM. *Breast Imaging: The Requisites*. Philadelphia: Elsevier Mosby, 2004:271-275.

History

▶ Calcifications detected on baseline screening mammogram. Magnification CC (craniocaudal) and ML (mediolateral) views are shown

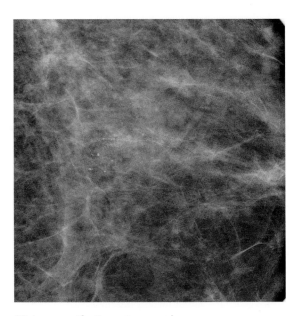

CC view, magnification mammography

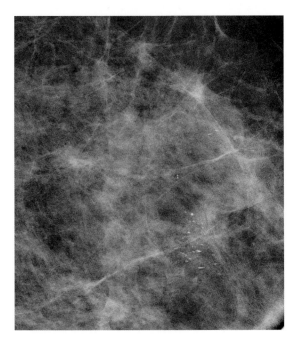

ML view, magnification mammography

Case 18   Milk of Calcium

Findings

- ► Grouped amorphous "smudgy" microcalcifications on the CC magnification view
- ► The 90-degree lateral magnification view clearly demonstrates layering ("teacup" appearance) of the same calcifications
  - ▪ Note the increased conspicuity on 90-degree lateral magnification view

Differential Diagnosis

- ► None—classic appearance demonstrated

Teaching Points

- ► Represents sedimented calcifications in small cysts
- ► Classically high-density calcium which changes shape between the CC and ML views
  - ▪ Indistinct, amorphous, circular/oval on CC view (*en face* view)
  - ▪ Assumes "teacup", semi-lunar, or meniscus appearance on 90-degree lateral
- ► Magnification views of calcifications permit better depiction of morphology
  - ▪ Beam must be directed horizontally (90 degrees) to calcifications
  - ▪ MLO magnification views will NOT optimally depict milk of calcium
  - ▪ Occasionally, leaving the patient in ML compression for 2 to 3 minutes will permit calcium to layer in the dependent portion of the microcysts and be more clearly depicted
- ► Calcium oxalate, which can manifest as microcalcifications on mammography requires polarized light microscopy for accurate identification by histology
- ► Beware the satisfaction of search
  - ▪ Malignant calcifications can coexist in patients with benign calcifications

Management

- ► BIRADS® Category 2: Benign findings
- ► Annual screening mammography

Selected References/Further Reading

American College of Radiology (ACR). ACR BI-RADS®—Mammography, 4th ed. *ACR Breast Imaging Reporting and Data Systems, Breast Imaging Atlas*. Reston, VA. American College of Radiology, 2003:80-84.

Bassett LW, et al. *Diagnosis of Diseases of the Breast*, 2nd ed. Philadelphia: WB Saunders Co., 2005:435.

Ikeda DM. *Breast Imaging: The Requisites*. Philadelphia: Elsevier Mosby, 2004:73-75.

History

▸ Screening mammogram (left breast images included)

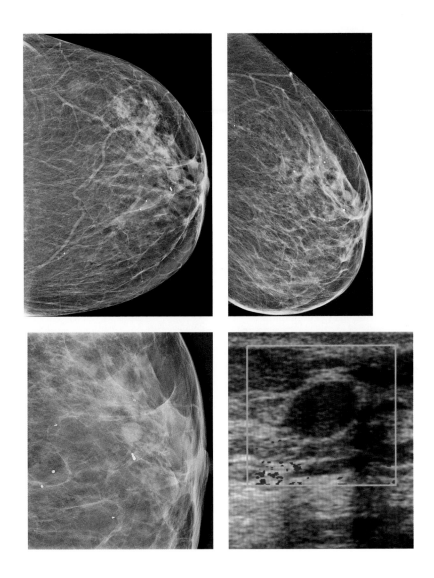

Case 19 Complicated Cyst

Findings

- Mammogram: There is a round-to-oval equal-density, circumscribed mass (*circles*) in the subareolar breast
- Ultrasound: There is a parallel, hypoechoic mass with posterior acoustic enhancement and no Doppler flow

Differential Diagnosis

- Simple cyst (with artifactual internal echoes)
- Galactocele
- Solid mass
  - Fibroadenoma
  - Mucinous carcinoma
- If thick wall, thick septations, and/or mural nodule/intracystic mass present, consider the differential for complex cyst
  - Intraductal papilloma
  - Intracyctic papillary DCIS
  - Invasive ductal carcinoma (high-grade IDC can be a circumscribed, nearly anechoic mass)

Teaching Points

- Commonly encountered
- *Complicated* cysts contain internal echoes that may or may not be mobile during real-time ultrasound scanning
  - May have a layered appearance (fluid/debris level)
  - May shift with changes in positioning
- The absence of blood flow is not a reliable discriminator for cystic versus solid masses as not all solid masses will demonstrate Doppler flow
- May be palpable/symptomatic or detected incidentally
- Most commonly seen in mid 40s to early 50s
- Frequently co-exist with simple cysts

Management

- If incidental/asymptomatic, and mobile internal echoes or fluid/debris level present, annual screening recommended
  - If atypical features, non-mobile echoes present, or concern that the mass is solid, then ultrasound-guided aspiration recommended
  - Non-bloody aspirate should be discarded as it is unreliable for diagnosis
- If new/enlarging or painful, ultrasound-guided aspiration/biopsy should be considered for diagnosis and/or symptomatic relief

Selected References/Further Readings

American College of Radiology (ACR). ACR BI-RADS®—Mammography, 4th ed. *ACR Breast Imaging Reporting and Data Systems, Breast Imaging Atlas*. Reston, VA. American College of Radiology, 2003:60-61.

Berg W, et al. *Diagnostic Imaging Breast*. Salt Lake City, UT: Amirsys Inc., 2006:35-39.

Stavros AT. *Breast Ultrasound*. Philadelphia: Lippincott Williams & Wilkins, 2004:276-350.

History

▶ Painful, erythematous mass in the left breast, upper outer quadrant. The patient reports malaise and low-grade fever for 2 days

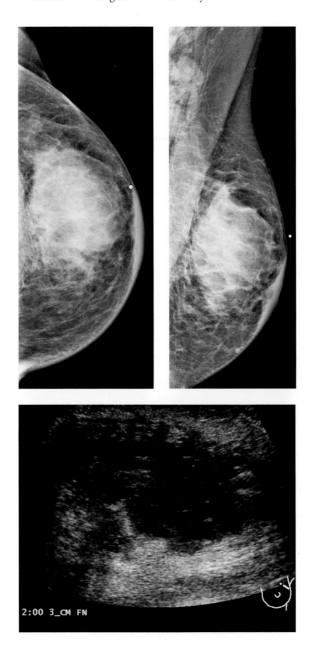

Case 20 Abscess

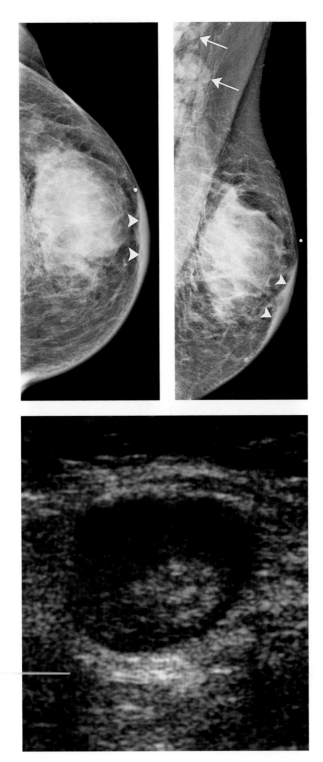

Axilla

Findings

► Mammogram
  ▪ Increased soft tissue density and an obscured mass at the 2 o'clock position (skin BB marker)
  ▪ Trabecular thickening, skin thickening (*arrowheads*), and axillary adenopathy (*arrows*)
► Ultrasound:
  ▪ Irregular, heterogeneously hypoechoic mass with a thickened rim and posterior acoustic enhancement
  ▪ During real-time scanning, some mobile internal debris was evident. An enlarged axillary lymph node correlates with the mammogram findings
► Clinical exam demonstrates marked erythema, skin thickening, and extreme tenderness

Differential Diagnosis

► High-grade invasive ductal carcinoma with features of inflammatory carcinoma

Teaching Points

► Begins as mastitis
► Most common organisms are *Streptococcus* and *Staphylococcus* entering through broken skin or nipple
► Typically subareolar but may be peripheral, as in this patient
► Ultrasound is the favored imaging modality in patients less than 30 years old
  ▪ Patients may not tolerate mammography due to pain
► Most common in lactating mothers (puerperal mastitis)
► May occur in immune-compromised or diabetic patients
► Chronic smokers may have recurrent subareolar abscess formation
  ▪ Can develop spontaneous periareolar fistulas

Management

► Culture (aspiration can be performed by palpation or using ultrasound guidance)
► Antibiotic therapy (oral or intravenous depending on size/organism)
► Larger abscesses may require indwelling catheter placement or surgical treatment
► Must follow up to complete clinical resolution to exclude underlying carcinoma

Selected References/Further Reading

Ikeda DM. *Breast Imaging: The Requisites*. Philadelphia: Elsevier Mosby, 2004:126-128.
Cardenosa G. *Clinical Breast Imaging: A Patient-Focused Teaching File*. Philadelphia: Lippincott Williams & Wilkins, 2007:395-397.
Stavros AT. *Breast Ultrasound*. Philadelphia: Lippincott Williams & Wilkins, 2004:361-393.

History

▶ Screening mammogram

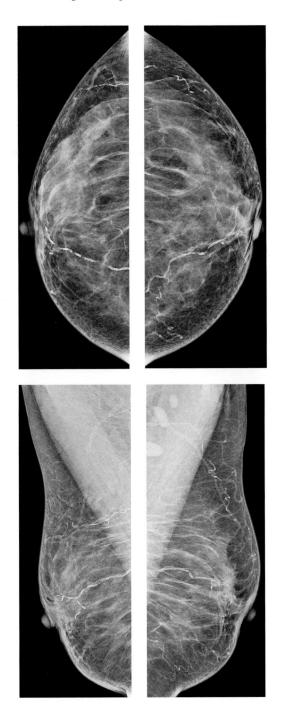

Case 21 Vascular Calcifications

Findings

▸ Mammogram: There are multiple dense, parallel ("tram-track") calcifications in tubular structures

Differential Diagnosis

▸ None—classic appearance demonstrated

Teaching Points

▸ Represents calcification within the arterial walls (atherosclerosis)
▸ Common, especially in diabetic and dialysis patients
▸ Increased frequency with advancing age
▸ Most cases easily recognized
▸ Magnification views may be helpful to delineate detail and confirm diagnosis when early or developing
▸ Look for a non-calcified portion of a vessel leading up to the calcification in order to differentiate from other causes of calcification
  ▪ When atypical imaging features are present consider
    ◆ Secretory calcifications
    ◆ Ductal carcinoma in situ (DCIS)

Management

▸ Annual screening mammography

Selected References/Further Reading

American College of Radiology (ACR). ACR BI-RADS®—Mammography, 4th ed. *ACR Breast Imaging Reporting and Data Systems, Breast Imaging Atlas*. Reston, VA: American College of Radiology, 2003:66-67.

Cardenosa G. *Clinical Breast Imaging: A Patient-Focused Teaching File*. Philadelphia: Lippincott Williams & Wilkins, 2007:117-118.

Ikeda DM. *Breast Imaging: The Requisites*. Philadelphia: Elsevier Mosby, 2004:81.

History

▶ Palpable mass left breast, upper outer quadrant (metallic BB)

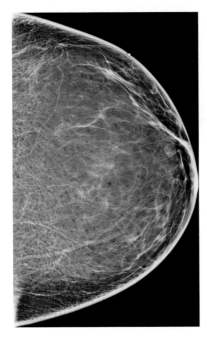
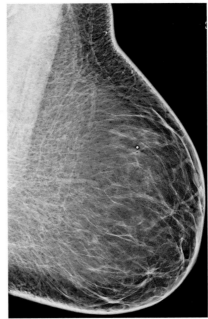

Case 22　Lipoma

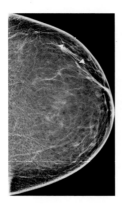 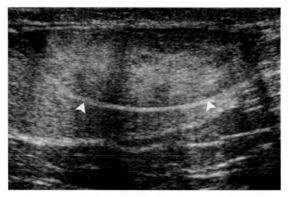

Findings

▶ Mammogram: Oval/lenticular, circumscribed, fat-density, superficial mass (*arrowheads*)
▶ Ultrasound: Parallel homogenous mass with echotexture identical to surrounding fat (*arrowheads*)
▶ Clinical exam demonstrates a non-tender, soft, mobile mass

Differential Diagnosis

▶ Classic appearance demonstrated
▶ Hamartoma (fibroadenolipoma) may mimic lipoma when scant fibroglandular elements are present

Teaching Points

▶ May occur anywhere in the breast
　▪ Most arise within the subcutaneous fat layer
　▪ Less often within the retroglandular fat
▶ Mammogram appearance
　▪ Radiolucent/fat-density mass with thin radiopaque capsule
　　♦ Capsule may or may not be visible
　▪ Tangent mammographic view may depict the mass to better advantage
▶ Ultrasound appearance
　▪ Ultrasound typically not warranted
　▪ Variable: isoechoic to mildly hyperechoic relative to adjacent fat lobules
　▪ Capsule may or may not be visible

Management

▶ BI-RADS® Category 2: Benign finding
▶ Annual screening mammography

Selected References/Further Reading

Bassett LW, et al. *Diagnosis of Diseases of the Breast*, 2nd ed. Philadelphia: WB Saunders Co., 2005:457-460.
Ikeda DM. *Breast Imaging: The Requisites*. Philadelphia: Elsevier Mosby, 2004:120-122.
Stavros AT. *Breast Ultrasound*. Philadelphia: Lippincott Williams & Wilkins, 2004:569-575.

History

► Screening mammogram (bilateral MLO images shown)

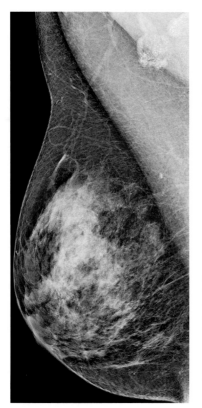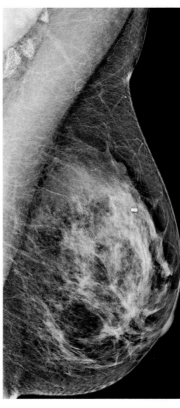

Case 23 Axillary Lymph Node Calcifications

Findings

▸ Hyperdensities (calcifications) are present in the axillary lymph nodes bilaterally

Differential Diagnosis

▸ Antiperspirant/deodorant artifact
▸ DDx for "hyperdensities" within axillary lymph node
  ▪ Granulomatous disease (histoplasmosis, tuberculosis, sarcoid)
  ▪ Silicone from prior implant rupture
  ▪ Metastatic disease (from breast, ovarian, or papillary thyroid primary)
  ▪ Gold particles from rheumatoid arthritis treatment (uncommon and of historical importance only)

Teaching Points

▸ Bilateral axillary nodal calcifications are most commonly due to granulomatous disease
  ▪ Usually coarse, dense with a benign appearance (as in this case)
▸ Silicone from extracapsular rupture of silicone breast implants can migrate into axillary lymph nodes
  ▪ Ruptured implant may be present or may have been explanted
    ♦ History of prior rupture/explantation usually provided
  ▪ May see adjacent "free" silicone in the breast
▸ Calcifications from metastatic malignancy may be unilateral or bilateral
  ▪ Ovarian metastasis calcifications are typically amorphous in morphology (reflect psammoma body formation)
  ▪ Calcifications from metastatic breast primary may appear similar to the primary tumor (e.g., pleomorphic)
    ♦ Careful inspection of the ipsilateral mammogram necessary

Management

▸ Recall from screening mammogram when there is an associated suspicious mammographic finding
▸ If there is a known history of granulomatous disease, then annual screening mammography is appropriate

Selected References/Further Readings

Cardenosa G. *Clinical Breast Imaging: A Patient-Focused Teaching File*. Philadelphia: Lippincott Williams & Wilkins, 2007:306.
Ikeda DM. *Breast Imaging: The Requisites*. Philadelphia: Elsevier Mosby, 2004:303-304.
Kopans DB. *Atlas of Breast Imaging*. Philadelphia: Lippincott Williams & Wilkins, 1999: 146-151.

History

► Screening mammogram (left breast images included)

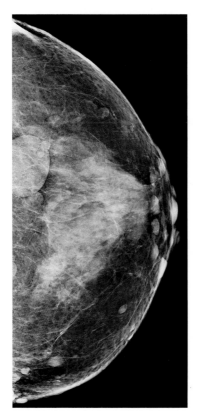
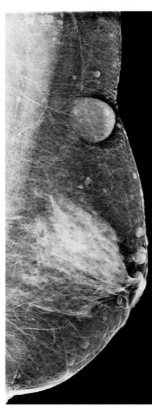

Case 24   Neurofibromatosis Type 1

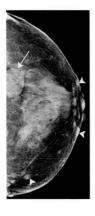 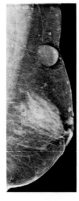

Findings

► Multiple masses of varying size project over the left breast on both views
► Note the sharp margin and air-crescent, or lucent "halo" (*arrow*) surrounding many of the lesions (*arrowheads*)

Differential Diagnosis

► None—classic appearance demonstrated

Teaching Points

► Autosomal dominant inheritance pattern
► Also known as von Recklinghausen's disease
► Accounts for 90% of neurofibromatosis patients
► Results in multiple, bilateral, raised skin lesions
  ▪ Lesions imaged in profile (tangent) will project from the skin
  ▪ Those projecting over the parenchyma will have sharp margins and a partial or complete air-crescent
► Can mimic a solid mass within the breast
  ▪ If uncertain, place a metallic marker over the lesion in question and perform a single tangent view
► Careful attention to the underlying parenchyma is critical to avoid overlooking a suspicious finding
► Commonly larger and more pronounced in the periareolar tissue
► The imaging technologist should document the presence of multiple raised skin lesions

Management

► Annual screening mammography

Selected References/Further Reading

Bassett LW, et al. *Diagnosis of Diseases of the Breast*, 2nd ed. Philadelphia: WB Saunders Co., 2005:401.
Cardenosa G. *Clinical Breast Imaging: A Patient-Focused Teaching File.* Philadelphia: Lippincott Williams & Wilkins, 2007:2-3.
Ikeda DM. *Breast Imaging: The Requisites.* Philadelphia: Elsevier Mosby, 2004:315.

History

▶ Decrease in left breast size

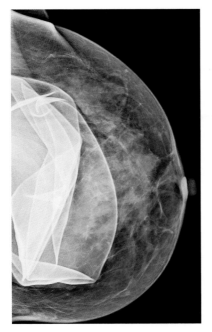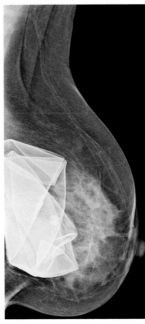

Case 25 Collapsed Saline Breast Implant

Findings

▶ Mammogram: Saline implant is collapsed; note the redundant folds and lack of volume on both views (appearance similar to a deflated balloon)

Differential Diagnosis

▶ Classic appearance demonstrated

Teaching Points

▶ Clinically, patient reports an abrupt change in the breast size/appearance
  ▪ Sometimes associated with blunt trauma
▶ Diagnosis of ruptured *saline* implant made clinically: Imaging is not required
  ▪ This patient was overdue for screening mammography and imaging was requested in advance of implant revision to exclude malignancy before an elective breast surgery
▶ *Silicone* implant rupture is frequently asymptomatic and may require imaging for diagnosis
  ▪ Ultrasound for extracapsular rupture
  ▪ Non-contrast MR for intra- or extracapsular rupture

Management

▶ Explantation and replacement as desired by the patient
▶ Annual screening mammography

Selected References/Further Reading

Middleton MS, McNamara MP. *Breast Implant Imaging*. Philadelphia: Lippincott Williams & Wilkins, 2003:190-193.

History

► 40-year-old woman with a palpable mass in the right breast. This is her baseline mammogram

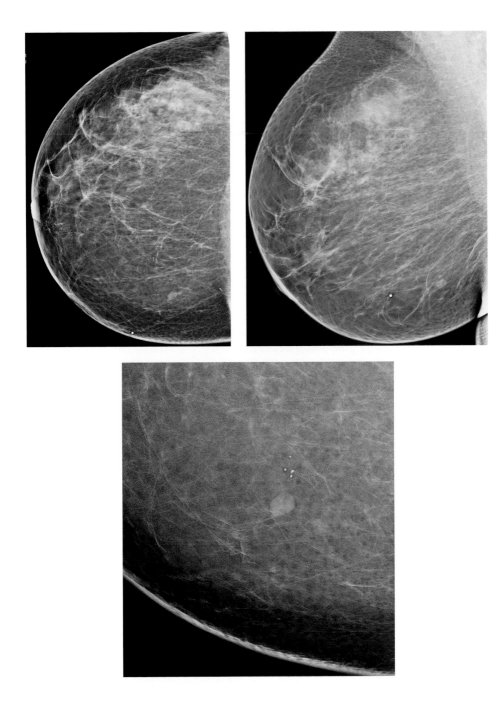

Case 26 Fibroadenoma

Findings

▶ A metallic BB denotes the palpable area of concern (note: BB not seen on magnification images)
▶ There is an oval, circumscribed, equal-density mass in the lower inner quadrant, corresponding with the palpable mass
▶ Benign calcifications are noted incidentally

Differential Diagnosis

▶ Lactating adenoma (in a pregnant or lactating female)
▶ Phyllodes tumor (when rapidly enlarging, or presenting as a larger mass)
▶ Tubular adenoma (rare)
▶ Malignancy (when atypical features are present, such as obscured or irregular margins)

Teaching Points

▶ Most common solid mass in women
  ▪ Peak incidence 20 to 30 years of age
▶ Multiple in 15% to 20% of patients
▶ When palpable, typically firm but mobile
  ▪ May fluctuate in size during menstrual cycle or pregnancy
▶ Mammogram: If classic "popcorn" or coarse calcifications are present, the mass is definitively benign and no further imaging is warranted
▶ Ultrasound: Classic appearance is a homogeneous, hypoechoic, parallel, circumscribed, oval, solid mass
  ▪ May or may not demonstrate posterior acoustic enhancement
  ▪ When degenerating, calcifications may cause posterior acoustic shadowing
  ▪ May not always demonstrate Doppler flow
▶ MR: Variable appearance, but frequently T2 intense, oval, circumscribed mass with homogeneous persistent enhancement
  ▪ May or may not demonstrate non-enhancing internal septations

Management

▶ Given the palpable presentation of this mass, ultrasound-guided core needle biopsy is recommended for tissue diagnosis (BI-RADS® Category 4A: Suspicious abnormality, low suspicion for malignancy)
▶ A *non-palpable* mass with similar imaging features (detected on a baseline screening mammogram) could be followed every six months until 2 years of stability was documented (BI-RADS® Category 3)
  ▪ BI-RADS® Category 3 assessment is reserved for non-palpable, non-calcified, well-circumscribed masses detected on baseline imaging (or in patients without available comparison exams) that have been subjected to a complete imaging evaluation
    ◆ BI-RADS® Category 3 assessment should *not* be assigned to a screening examination

Selected References/Further Reading

American College of Radiology (ACR). ACR BI-RADS®—Mammography, 4th ed. *ACR Breast Imaging Reporting and Data Systems, Breast Imaging Atlas*. Reston, VA: American College of Radiology, 2003:254, 258.
Bassett LW, et al. *Diagnosis of Diseases of the Breast*, 2nd ed. Philadelphia: WB Saunders Co., 2005:424-430.
Ikeda DM. *Breast Imaging: The Requisites*. Philadelphia: Elsevier Mosby, 2004:110-111.

History

▶ Screening mammogram

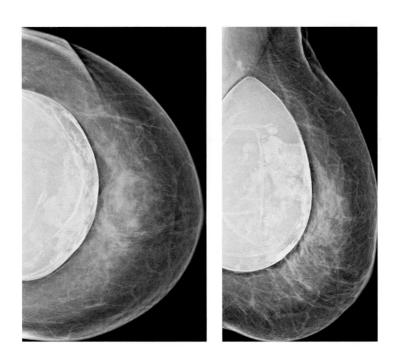

Case 27 Implant Capsular Calcifications

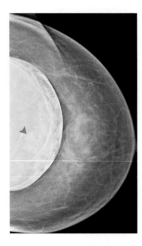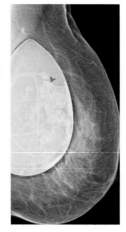

Findings

▶ Extensive plaque-like calcifications involve the fibrous capsule of the subglandular saline implant (*arrowheads* indicate representative areas)

Differential Diagnosis

▶ None—classic appearance demonstrated

Teaching Points

▶ Fibrous ("biological") capsules develop around implants shortly after implantation
  ▪ Imperceptible unless calcifications develop
▶ Capsular calcifications are common and benign
  ▪ Most frequent with implants more than 10 years old
▶ Classic appearance easily recognized
  ▪ Dystrophic, "sheet-like" or "plaque-like"
  ▪ Parallel and contiguous with the implant surface
  ▪ Can be visualized on standard and implant displaced views
  ▪ Magnification views should be performed if calcifications are suspected to arise from parenchyma
▶ Can be erroneously mistaken for extracapsular rupture
▶ May persist after explantation of subglandular implants without capsulectomy
  ▪ Calcifications remain just anterior to the pectoralis muscle
  ▪ Dense, linear, and "plaque-like"

Management

▶ Annual screening mammography

Selected References/Further Reading

Bassett LW, et al. *Diagnosis of Diseases of the Breast*, 2nd ed. Philadelphia: WB Saunders Co., 2005:604-607.

Ikeda DM. *Breast Imaging: The Requisites*. Philadelphia: Elsevier Mosby, 2004:252-262.

Middleton MS, McNamara MP. *Breast Implant Imaging*. Philadelphia: Lippincott Williams & Wilkins, 2003:284-285.

History

▶ Screening mammogram (and subsequent diagnostic ultrasound)

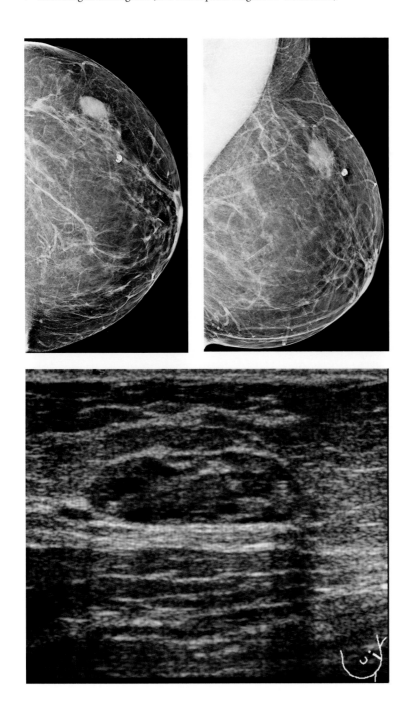

Case 28 Pseudoangiomatous Stromal Hyperplasia (PASH)

Findings

- ▶ Mammogram: Circumscribed, non-calcified, heterogeneous oval mass in the left upper outer quadrant
- ▶ Ultrasound: Parallel, mixed echogenicity, oval, circumscribed, solid mass without posterior acoustic enhancement or posterior acoustic shadowing

Differential Diagnosis

- ▶ Fibroadenoma
- ▶ Fibroadenolipoma/hamartoma
- ▶ Stromal fibrosis
- ▶ Phyllodes tumor

Teaching Points

- ▶ Typically incidental finding detected at screening mammography
  - ▪ Similar imaging features to fibroadenoma
  - ▪ Rarely may have architectural distortion or features suspicious for malignancy
- ▶ Can present as firm, painless palpable mass, or as local increased stroma
- ▶ Benign overgrowth of stromal tissue
  - ▪ Not considered premalignant or high-risk
- ▶ More common in premenopausal females
- ▶ Fine-needle aspiration nonspecific; core needle biopsy required for definitive diagnosis
  - ▪ Pathologist must distinguish PASH from low-grade angiosarcoma and phyllodes tumor
- ▶ Common incidental finding at core needle biopsy

Management

- ▶ Core needle biopsy recommended if palpable or enlarging or atypical imaging features at baseline presentation (e.g., angular margins)
- ▶ Return to annual screening mammography when core needle biopsy is benign and concordant
  - ▪ Larger masses may require excision

Selected References/Further Reading

Berg W, et al. *Diagnostic Imaging of the Breast*. Salt Lake City, UT: Amirsys Inc., 2006:66-69.
Celliers L, et al. Pseudoangiomatous stromal hyperplasia: a study of the mammographic and sonographic features. *Clin Radiol* 2010:65:145-149.
Stavros AT. *Breast Ultrasound*. Philadelphia: Lippincott Williams & Wilkins, 2004:581-584.

History

► 58 year-old woman with a palpable mass (indicated by a metallic BB) in the left breast, upper outer quadrant

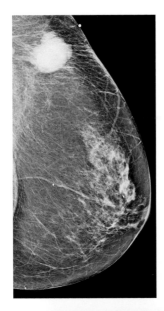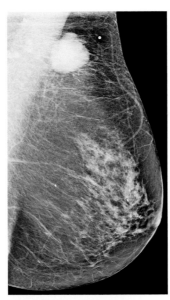

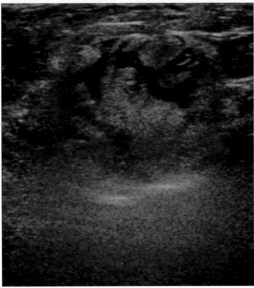

Case 29 Sarcoma

Findings

- Mammogram: High-density, round, non-calcified mass with circumscribed margins anteriorly, and somewhat ill-defined margins posteriorly. Note the mild lobulation superiorly
- Ultrasound: Round mass with indistinct margins and heterogeneous echogenicity

Differential Diagnosis

- Metastatic lymph node (given the upper outer quadrant location in this case)
- Invasive ductal carcinoma
- Phyllodes tumor

Teaching Points

- Rare
- Various types described (angiosarcoma, phyllodes tumor, liposarcoma, osteosarcoma)
  - May contain fibrous or osseous elements
  - Coarse calcifications may develop with osseous elements
- Frequently present as a palpable, painless, and rapidly enlarging mass
- May arise from breast or chest wall
  - Ultrasound or contrast-enhanced MR may help delineate origin
- Angiosarcoma may arise as a fast-growing vascular mass after breast irradiation
  - Highly malignant
- Poor prognosis for many of the types, depending on the grade

Management

- Core needle biopsy for tissue diagnosis
- Mastectomy versus wide local excision for definitive surgical therapy
- Staging evaluation
  - Hematogenous spread: metastasizes to the lung, bone, and liver
  - Lymph node metastases are rare; therefore, axillary lymph node dissection not usually indicated

Selected References/Further Reading

Bassett LW, et al. *Diagnosis of Diseases of the Breast*, 2nd ed. Philadelphia: WB Saunders Co., 2005:510-512.

Bland K, Copeland E. *The Breast: Comprehensive Management of Benign and Malignant Disorders*. St. Louis, MO: Saunders, 2004: Chapter 14.

Ikeda DM. *Breast Imaging: The Requisites*. Philadelphia: Elsevier Mosby, 2004:305.

History

▶ 53 year-old woman with left breast swelling and erythema

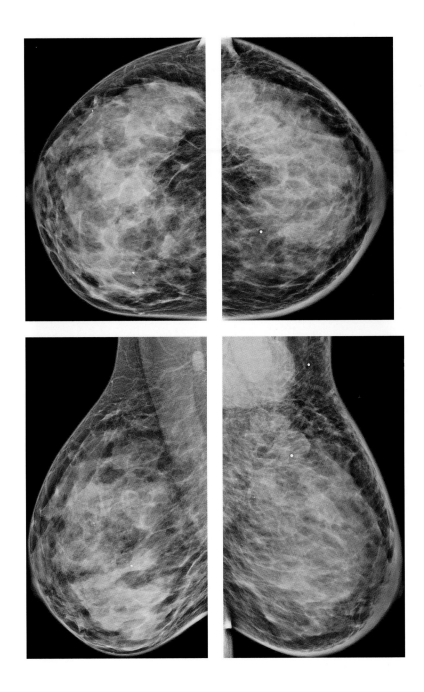

Case 30 Inflammatory Breast Carcinoma

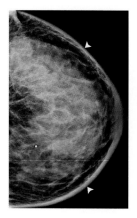 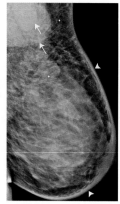 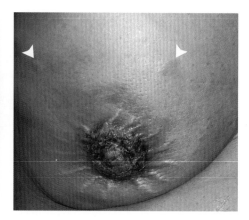

Findings

▶ Mammogram: Diffuse skin thickening (*arrowheads*), increased trabecular markings, and overall hazy (or "whiter") appearance, due to edema and decreased compressibility of the breast
  ▪ Large axillary lymph nodes are present (*arrows*)
▶ Photograph (from another patient) demonstrates clinical findings of erythema, *peau d'orange*, edema
  ▪ Note the raised erythematous lesions (*arrowheads*)
  ▪ There is tissue breakdown and discharge adjacent to the nipple (not a typical feature)

Differential Diagnosis

▶ Mastitis
▶ Mastitis complicated by abscess
▶ When unilateral breast edema is present, consider the following (unlikely in this particular case given the presence of adenopathy)
  ▪ Previous breast conservation/radiation therapy
  ▪ Trauma
  ▪ Venous obstruction (in the setting of an indwelling catheter)
  ▪ Asymmetric edema from congestive heart failure due to preferential positioning (i.e., sleeping on one side)

Teaching Points

▶ Rare, accounts for approximately 1% of all breast cancers
▶ Mammogram findings are variable (classic findings shown in this case) and may also include
  ▪ Breast mass
  ▪ Nipple retraction
  ▪ Focal asymmetry
  ▪ Suspicious microcalcifications (uncommon)
▶ Usually a clinical diagnosis

- ► Ultrasound demonstrates skin thickening and edema
  - ▪ Lower-frequency transducer may improve penetration
  - ▪ In few patients, may detect underlying mass
    - ◆ Often large and multifocal
  - ▪ May help direct biopsy
- ► "Punch" skin biopsy demonstrates tumor cells invading the dermal lymphatics
- ► Aggressive, with poor prognosis

Management

- ► Diagnosis with "punch" skin biopsy and/or ultrasound-guided core needle breast biopsy
- ► If there is high clinical suspicion for mastitis, a brief course of antibiotic therapy may be considered; however, biopsy should be performed if no clinical improvement is documented in 2 to 3 weeks
- ► Multimodal therapy including mastectomy, chemotherapy, and radiation may improve survival
  - ▪ Neoadjuvant chemotherapy is increasingly utilized as first-line treatment

Selected References/Further Reading

Bassett LW, et al. *Diagnosis of Diseases of the Breast*, 2nd ed. Philadelphia: WB Saunders Co., 2005:483-489.
Ikeda DM. *Breast Imaging: The Requisites*. Philadelphia: Elsevier Mosby, 2004:296-302.
Stavros AT. *Breast Ultrasound*. Philadelphia: Lippincott Williams & Wilkins, 2004:676-680.

History

► Abnormal screening mammogram (diagnostic mammogram images shown)

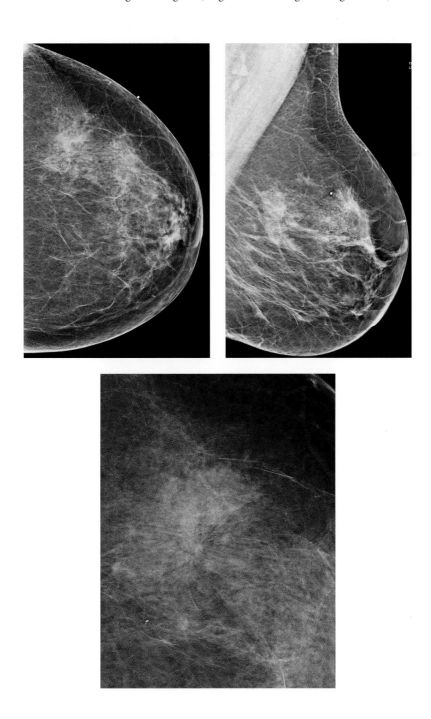

Case 31 Radial Scar

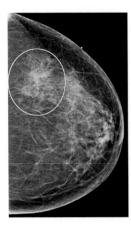 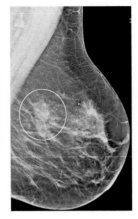 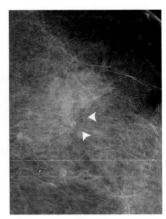

Findings

- ▶ Architectural distortion in the upper outer quadrant (*circles*)
- ▶ Note the long spicules, and relative central lucency (*arrowheads*) on the spot magnification view

Differential Diagnosis

- ▶ Invasive ductal carcinoma
- ▶ Invasive lobular carcinoma
- ▶ Tubular carcinoma
- ▶ Architectural distortion from prior lumpectomy/biopsy

Teaching Points

- ▶ Benign lesion that can simulate malignancy mammographically
  - ▪ Despite the term "scar," it is *not* the result of prior trauma or surgery
- ▶ Classic mammographic features shown but may also demonstrate:
  - ▪ Central density
  - ▪ Associated microcalcifications
- ▶ Nonspecific and variable ultrasound appearance
  - ▪ Ranges from non-apparent to an ill-defined, hypoechoic mass to a shadowing irregular mass with features similar to invasive ductal carcinoma
- ▶ May have associated atypical ductal hyperplasia, low-grade DCIS or tubular carcinoma
- ▶ Has multiple synonyms in the literature and in practice
  - ▪ Complex sclerosing lesion, radial sclerosing lesion, non-encapsulated sclerosing lesion
  - ▪ Pathologists may differentiate terminology based on size
    - ◆ <1 cm: radial scar
    - ◆ >1 cm: complex sclerosing lesion
- ▶ Usually an incidental, asymptomatic finding

Management

► Biopsy is warranted
  ▪ Radial scar cannot be distinguished from malignancy based on imaging
► Controversy exists over method of biopsy
  ▪ Percutaneous core needle biopsy (PCNB) versus excisional biopsy when radial scar is the favored diagnosis
  ▪ PCNB can be performed; however, surgical excision is usually recommended when radial scar is found at core biopsy
    ◆ Reports of associated or adjacent malignancy
    ◆ May be under-sampling with PCNB

Further Readings/Selected References

Bassett LW, et al. *Diagnosis of Diseases of the Breast*, 2nd ed. Philadelphia: WB Saunders Co., 2005:449-451.

Stavros AT. *Breast Ultrasound*. Philadelphia: Lippincott Williams & Wilkins, 2004:703-709.

Tabar L, et al. *Breast Cancer: The Art and Science of Early Detection with Mammography*. New York: Thieme, 2005:392-393.

History

▶ Screening mammogram

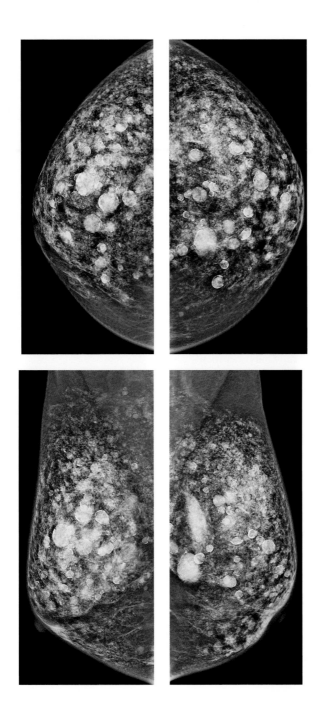

Case 32   Direct Silicone Injections

Findings

▸ Innumerable high-density round masses with "eggshell" calcifications throughout both breasts (silicone granulomas)

Differential Diagnosis

▸ None—classic appearance demonstrated
- Paraffin injections can have a similar appearance

Teaching Points

▸ Breast augmentation with various injected substances, including paraffin, was first documented in the early 1900s
- Silicone injections were first reported in Japan in 1946
▸ Silicone was frequently contaminated or adulterated
▸ Reported complications include disfigurement, granuloma formation, migration, pulmonary emboli, and rarely death
▸ Coalescence of the liquid silicone forms masses called oleomas
- Become palpable
- Mammography can confirm silicone granuloma
▸ Significantly limits physical exam reducing the ability to detect a clinically significant mass
▸ Substantially reduces sensitivity of screening mammography
- Renders mammography almost useless for the detection of early malignancy in certain patients
▸ Ultrasound demonstrates a "snowstorm" appearance
- Obscures underlying tissue and limits evaluation
▸ Illegal practice in the United States
▸ Still performed in parts of Asia

Management

▸ Counsel patients regarding limitations of mammography and ultrasound imaging for breast cancer screening
▸ Contrast-enhanced MR may be considered for screening, given reduced sensitivity of mammography and ultrasound
- Granulomas may enhance, confounding imaging and interpretation

Selected References/Further Reading

Bassett LW, et al. *Diagnosis of Diseases of the Breast*, 2nd ed. Philadelphia: WB Saunders Co., 2005:601-602.

Berg W, et al. *Diagnostic Imaging of the Breast*. Salt Lake City, UT: Amirsys Inc., 2006: Part IV, Chapter 4, 2-5.

Middleton MS, McNamara MP. *Breast Implant Imaging*. Philadelphia: Lippincott Williams & Wilkins, 2003:2-8 and 272-282.

History

► 37-year-old woman with a tender, palpable, tubular mass in the right breast

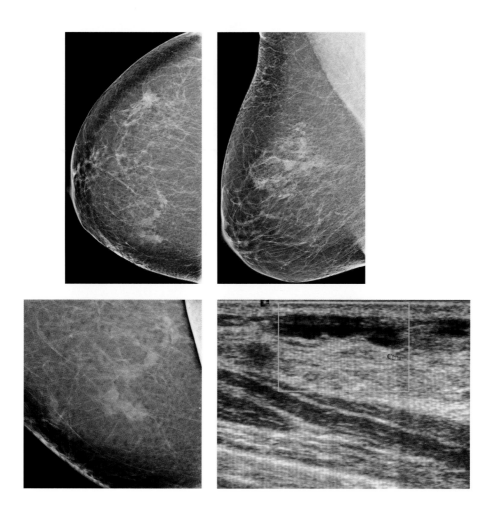

Case 33   Mondor Disease (Also Known as Mondor's Disease)

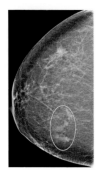
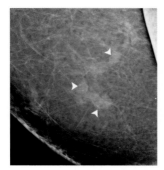
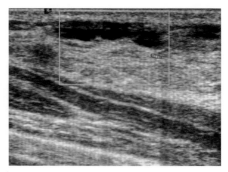

Findings

▶ The palpable mass corresponds with a superficial, dilated, tubular hypoechoic/anechoic structure with no demonstrable flow by color Doppler (*circled* on full view; *arrowheads* on magnification view)

Differential Diagnosis

▶ Dilated duct

Teaching Points

▶ Uncommon
▶ Benign superficial thrombophlebitis of the thoracoepigastric, lateral thoracic, or superior epigastric vein
▶ Classically presents as a palpable cord (with or without associated tenderness)
▶ Typically occurs in younger patients (third to fifth decade)
▶ Incidence: women > men (3:1)
▶ Most cases are idiopathic, self-limiting, and inconsequential
▶ Chronic thrombophlebitis may result in vascular calcifications
▶ Rare association with underlying breast malignancy, mammography should be performed in patients over age 35

Management

▶ Symptomatic treatment and reassurance; most cases resolve in several weeks

Selected References/Further Reading

Bassett LW, et al. *Diagnosis of Diseases of the Breast*, 2nd ed. Philadelphia: WB Saunders Co., 2005:405-407.

Conant EF, Wilkes AN, Mendelson EB, Feig SA. Superficial thrombophlebitis of the breast (Mondor disease): Mammographic findings. *AJR* 1993;160:1201-1203.

Shetty MK, et al. Mondor's disease of the breast; sonographic and mammographic findings. *AJR* 2001;177:893-896.

History

► Abnormal screening mammogram; magnification views of calcifications shown

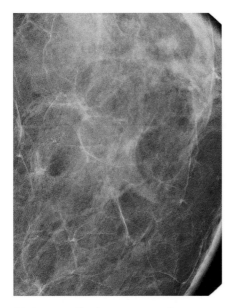

CC view, magnification mammography

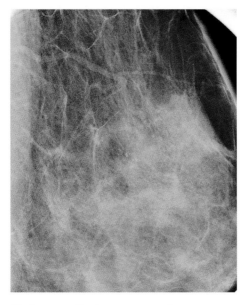

ML view, magnification mammography

Case 34 Atypical Ductal Hyperplasia (ADH)

Findings

► Grouped amorphous (indistinct) calcifications

Differential Diagnosis

► Low-grade ductal carcinoma in situ (DCIS)
► Usual ductal hyperplasia
► Fibrocystic change

Teaching Points

► ADH is most often found in association with amorphous calcifications
  ▪ 20% of biopsies for amorphous calcifications will contain ADH
► Pathologically, defined as having some but not all of the features of low-grade DCIS
  ▪ Nuclei may appear enlarged, irregular, and hyperchromatic
  ▪ Can be difficult for pathologist to distinguish ADH from DCIS with core needle biopsy samples
► ADH on core biopsy warrants excisional biopsy
  ▪ Variable reports of upgrade to malignancy (DCIS or invasive carcinoma)
    ◆ 10% to 25% in large-core biopsy patients
► High-risk marker for breast cancer
  ▪ Four- to five-fold increased relative risk
  ▪ Risk increased bilaterally

Management

► Tissue diagnosis of microcalcifications with vacuum-assisted stereotactic core needle biopsy (CNB)
► While ADH found at CNB requires surgical excision, re-excision is not required when present at the margins of a surgical specimen
► ADH as the only risk factor for breast cancer should not prompt screening MR
  ▪ With other risk factors, if calculated lifetime risk exceeds 20%, consider MR screening
► Consider chemoprevention (tamoxifen)

Selected References/Further Reading

Berg WA. Image-guided breast biopsy and management of high-risk lesions. *Radiol Clin North Am* 2004;42(5):935-946.

Berg WA, et al. Biopsy of amorphous breast calcifications: Pathologic outcome and yield at stereotactic biopsy. *Radiology* 2001;221:495-503.

Ikeda DM. *Breast Imaging: The Requisites*. Philadelphia: Elsevier Mosby, 2004:183-184.

History

▶ 35-year-old woman with several firm, palpable masses in the right breast. The masses developed several months after a motor vehicle accident. Tangent magnification mammography images shown

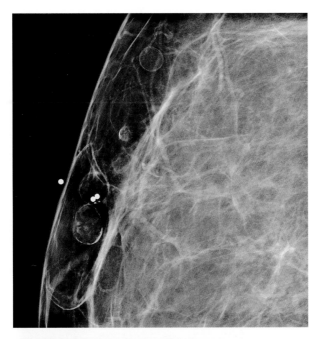

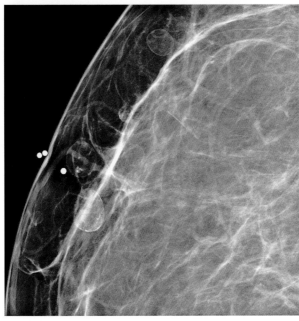

Case 35   Oil Cysts/Fat Necrosis from a Seat-Belt Injury

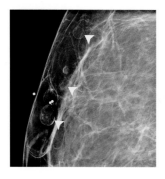 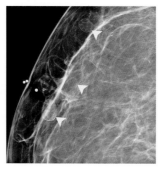

Findings

▶ Metallic BBs mark the palpable areas of concern. There are multiple round and oval, circumscribed, fat-density masses with varying degrees of peripheral, "eggshell" calcifications (*arrowheads*)

Differential Diagnosis

▶ None—classic appearance of oil cysts demonstrated

Teaching Points

▶ Fat necrosis may result following any trauma to the breast:
  ▪ Blunt trauma
  ▪ Surgery (reduction mammoplasty, lumpectomy, reconstruction [e.g., TRAM flap])
▶ In motor vehicle accidents, the site of breast injury often correlates with seat-belt position
  ▪ May also reflect injury from airbag deployment
▶ Timing of injury helpful to correlate with imaging findings
  ▪ Acute: Breast hematoma
  ▪ Several months: Oil cysts possible
  ▪ Years: Dystrophic parenchymal calcifications possible
▶ Mammography is the preferred imaging modality
  ▪ Magnified tangent view is helpful to characterize oil cysts and confirm diagnosis
▶ Ultrasound often yields a variable and sometimes ominous appearance
  ▪ May depict non-specific, round, circumscribed hypoechoic or anechoic masses

Management

▶ BI-RADS® Category 2: Benign findings
▶ Reassure patient
▶ Annual screening mammography beginning at age 40

Selected References/Further Reading

DiPiro PJ, et al. Seat belt injuries of the breast: findings on mammography and sonography. *AJR* 1995;164:317-320.
Stavros AT. *Breast Ultrasound*. Philadelphia: Lippincott Williams & Wilkins, 2004:415-428.

History

► 43-year-old woman with a rapidly enlarging palpable mass in the right breast

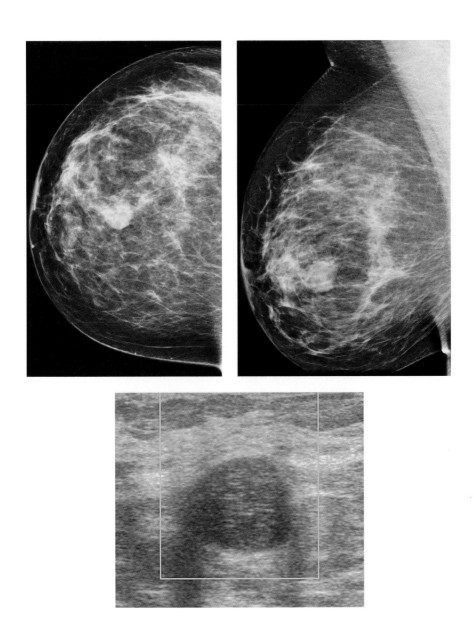

Case 36   Phyllodes Tumor

Findings

▸ Mammogram: Round, equal-density, non-calcified mass with partially obscured margins
▸ Ultrasound: Round, heterogenously hypoechoic mass with relatively circumscribed margins and associated posterior acoustic enhancement

Differential Diagnosis

▸ Fibroadenoma
▸ Invasive ductal carcinoma

Teaching Points

▸ Rare (<1% of all breast tumors)
  ▪ Peak incidence 45 to 49 years
▸ Similar imaging features to fibroadenoma
  ▪ Many cases demonstrate increased vascularity
▸ Is *not* a "giant fibroadenoma" (a term that should not be used)
▸ Commonly presents as a rapidly enlarging palpable mass
▸ Pathologically can be benign, locally aggressive or malignant
  ▪ Most are benign
  ▪ Larger tumors (>3 cm) more likely to be malignant
▸ *Phyllodes* means "leaf-like" which describes the stromal growth pattern

Management

▸ Ultrasound-guided core needle biopsy for diagnosis
  ▪ May be difficult for pathologist to distinguish from fibroadenoma
    ◆ If concerned, recommend excision
▸ If diagnosis of phyllodes confirmed, wide local excision recommended
  ▪ Radiation therapy reduces local recurrence
▸ Malignant variety spreads hematogenously (similar to sarcomas)
  ▪ Therefore, axillary lymph node sampling not usually required

Selected References/Further Reading

Bassett LW, et al. *Diagnosis of Diseases of the Breast*, 2nd ed. Philadelphia: WB Saunders Co., 2005:456-457.
Liberman L, et al. Benign and malignant phyllodes tumors: mammographic and sonographic findings. *Radiology* 1996;198:121-124.
Stavros AT. *Breast Ultrasound*. Philadelphia: Lippincott Williams & Wilkins, 2004:695-700.

History

▸ 51-year-old woman with a palpable mass detected by her new physician on routine clinical breast exam. The patient has a history of end-stage renal disease. The palpable mass is marked with a metallic BB

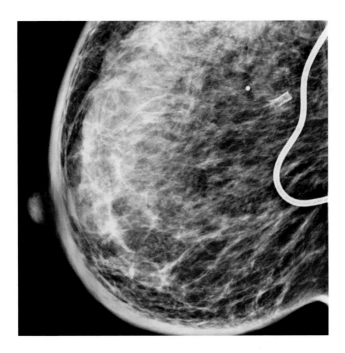

Case 37 Retained Catheter Cuff

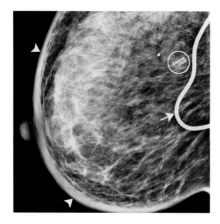

Findings

▶ The palpable mass corresponds with a retained cuff from a previous central venous catheter (*circled*)

▶ A portion of a separate, current hemodialysis catheter is also included on the film (*arrow*)

▶ Note also diffuse skin thickening; this is secondary to edema from chronic fluid overload (*arrowheads*)

Differential Diagnosis

▶ None—classic findings demonstrated

Teaching Points

▶ Most tunneled central venous catheters (used for long-term venous access, including hemodialysis) have a polyester (Dacron) cuff. Fibrous tissue growth is stimulated by the cuff to anchor the catheter

▶ Cuffs are removed via traction or blunt dissection when the catheter is no longer required or has become infected

▶ Retention of catheter cuffs has been widely reported

▶ Catheter cuff retention is typically inconsequential

▶ Usually noted in the upper inner quadrant of the right breast

▶ May present as a firm, palpable mass
  ▪ More commonly found incidentally on a screening mammogram

Management

▶ In the absence of infection, no action is required

▶ Annual screening mammography

Selected References/Further Reading

Beyer GA, et al. Mammographic appearance of the retained Dacron cuff of a Hickman catheter. *AJR* 1990;155:1203-1204.

Ellis RL, et al. Mammography of breasts in which the catheter cuffs have been retained: normal, infected and postoperative appearances. *AJR* 1997;169:713-715.

Ikeda DM. *Breast Imaging: The Requisites*. Philadelphia: Elsevier Mosby, 2004:314-315.

History

▶ Screening mammogram

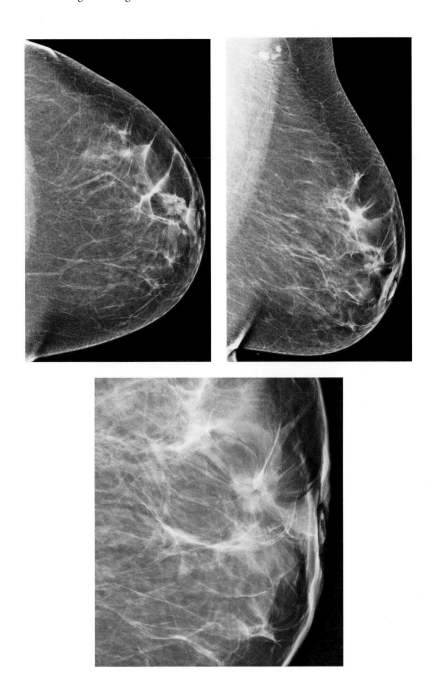

Case 38 Invasive Lobular Carcinoma with Nipple Retraction

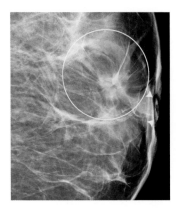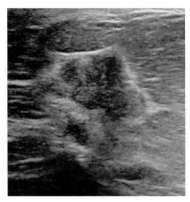

Findings

▶ Mammogram: Architectural distortion with the suggestion of a lobular mass with spiculated margins in the subareolar breast. The spot magnification image shows margin detail to greatest advantage (*circle*)
  ▪ Note the associated nipple retraction (*arrowheads*)
▶ Ultrasound: Lobular, hypoechoic mass with angular margins and posterior acoustic shadowing

Differential Diagnosis

▶ Invasive ductal carcinoma
▶ Postoperative scar

Teaching Points

▶ Nipple *retraction* should be distinguished from benign nipple *inversion*
  ▪ Benign nipple inversion
    ◆ Often long-standing and bilateral
    ◆ Can be corrected (everted) with manual pressure
  ▪ Nipple retraction
    ◆ Malignancy can result in thickening and shortening of subareolar ducts
    ◆ New or increasing retraction should prompt thorough evaluation for underlying malignancy
▶ Imaging pitfalls
  ▪ Subareolar masses may be difficult to perceive mammographically
    ◆ Nipples must be profiled on at least one view (screening exams)
    ◆ Perform spot magnification views with nipple in profile when patient presents for diagnostic evaluation
  ▪ Ultrasound of subareolar tissue must be performed carefully
    ◆ Nipple areolar complex normally shadows
    ◆ May need to angle beam to best visualize tissue
▶ Presentation and clinical course
  ▪ Skin/nipple retraction may be postoperative
    ◆ Correlate with prior scars and use mammographic scar markers if necessary

- Rarely, patient may report bloody or serous nipple discharge
- Cancers in this location may metastasize to the lymph nodes early
  - Use ultrasound to evaluate the axilla for possible lymph node metastasis

Management

▶ Ultrasound-guided core needle biopsy for tissue diagnosis
▶ When diagnosis confirmed, consider MR to evaluate extent of disease and for ancillary screening of the contralateral breast

Selected References/Further Reading

Bassett LW, et al. *Diagnosis of Diseases of the Breast*, 2nd ed. Philadelphia: WB Saunders Co., 2005:488-489.
Stavros AT. *Breast Ultrasound*. Philadelphia: Lippincott Williams & Wilkins, 2004:560-569.
Tabar L, et al. *Breast Cancer: The Art and Science of Early Detection with Mammography*. New York: Thieme, 2005:423-428.

History

▶ 26-year-old woman who is 39 weeks pregnant with a mobile, soft, palpable mass

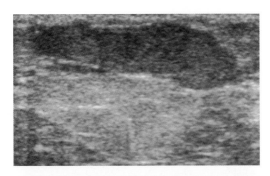

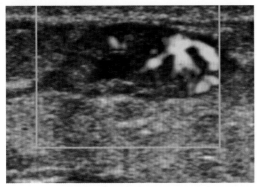

Case 39 Lactating Adenoma

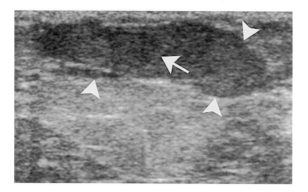

Findings

- Ultrasound: Circumscribed oval, parallel, mass (*arrowheads*) with heterogeneous echotexture and internal septa (*arrow*)
  - Increased vascularity on color Doppler

Differential Diagnosis

- Fibroadenoma
- Invasive ductal carcinoma

Teaching Points

- Benign tumor, related to fibroadenoma and tubular adenoma
- Most commonly present in third trimester or during lactation
- New palpable masses in pregnant and lactating patients are common
  - Must be carefully evaluated to exclude malignancy
- Classic imaging findings: circumscribed, homogenously hypoechoic mass with parallel orientation and posterior acoustic enhancement; typically 2 to 4 cm
  - Similar imaging features to fibroadenoma
  - May be multiple
  - But may mimic malignancy when angular margins or internal heterogeneity are present
- Most regress after cessation of breast feeding

Management

- Ultrasound-guided core needle biopsy
  - Consent for the possibility of a milk fistula
    - Rare and less likely with core needle biopsy than excisional biopsy
  - Fine-needle aspiration may not be diagnostic

Selected References/Further Reading

Berg W, et al. *Diagnostic Imaging of the Breast*. Salt Lake City, UT: Amirsys Inc., 2006: Part IV, Chapter 5, 12-15.
Stavros AT. *Breast Ultrasound*. Philadelphia: Lippincott Williams & Wilkins, 2004:554-560.
Sumkin, JH et al. Lactating adenoma: US features and literature review. *Radiology* 1998;206:271-274.

History

► 62-year-old male with a palpable right breast mass

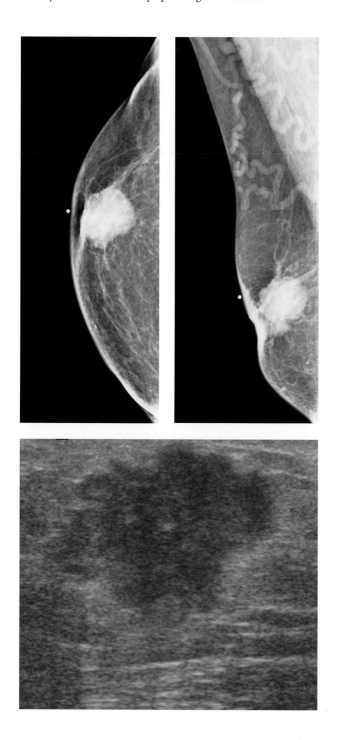

Case 40   Male Breast Cancer (Invasive Ductal Carcinoma)

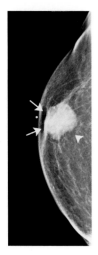 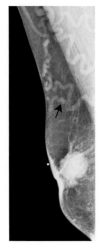 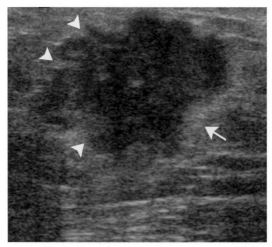

Findings

▶ Mammogram: Dense lobular mass with minimally spiculated margins (*arrowhead*) with associated nipple retraction and skin thickening (*arrows*)
  ▪ Note the engorged vessels (*black arrow*)
▶ Ultrasound: Irregular, heterogeneously hypoechoic solid mass with microlobulated margins (*arrowheads*) and an echogenic rim (*arrow*)

Differential Diagnosis

▶ None—classic appearance demonstrated
▶ In male patients with a palpable mass, consider gynecomastia (but imaging excludes gynecomastia in this case)

Teaching Points

▶ Rare (<1% of all breast cancers)
▶ Classic mammogram findings: subareolar, high-density, lobulated mass with spiculated margins (similar features to IDC in women)
  ▪ Distinguish from the "flame shape" of gynecomastia
    ◆ Extensive gynecomastia can obscure underlying mass
  ▪ Calcifications uncommon
  ▪ Intracystic papillary DCIS may have circumscribed margins
▶ Ultrasound typically demonstrates irregular hypoechoic shadowing mass
▶ Clinically presents as a non-tender, firm palpable mass
  ▪ Nipple retraction more common (compared to female patients)
  ▪ Mean age 60 to 64 years
  ▪ 50% have palpable adenopathy at presentation
  ▪ Serous or bloody nipple discharge possible
▶ Overwhelmingly male breast cancer is invasive ductal carcinoma (85%)
  ▪ Other histologic subtypes are unusual

Management

► Ultrasound-guided core needle biopsy for tissue diagnosis
  ▪ If suspicious axillary lymph nodes are present, tissue-sampling with ultrasound-guided fine-needle aspiration or core needle biopsy may confirm metastatic disease
► Perform contralateral mammogram to exclude occult malignancy (uncommon)
► Refer patient for genetic counseling
  ▪ Approximately 10% will have a BRCA2 gene mutation

Selected References/Further Reading

Cardenosa G. *Clinical Breast Imaging: A Patient-Focused Teaching File*. Philadelphia: Lippincott Williams & Wilkins, 2007:326-327.
Dershaw DD, et al. Mammographic findings in men with breast cancer. *AJR* 1993;160:267-270.
Stavros AT. *Breast Ultrasound*. Philadelphia: Lippincott Williams & Wilkins, 2004:732-739.

History

▶ 61-year-old woman with a new palpable mass in the left breast. Mammogram obtained 8 months ago (not shown) was normal

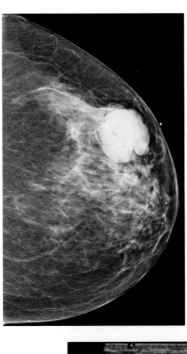
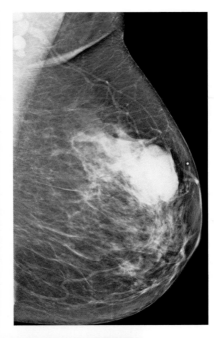

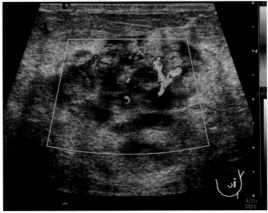

Case 41   Primary Breast Lymphoma (B-cell)

Findings

- ► Mammogram
  - ▪ Lobular, high-density, circumscribed mass
  - ▪ Several dense lymph nodes are present in the left axilla on the MLO view
- ► Ultrasound
  - ▪ Heterogeneous, irregular, hypervascular mass with indistinct margins and posterior acoustic enhancement

Differential Diagnosis

- ► Invasive ductal carcinoma
- ► Metastatic lymphoma or other non-breast primary malignancy

Teaching Points

- ► Rare (<0.6% of all breast malignancies)
  - ▪ Diagnosis not usually considered unless patient has a history of lymphoma (treated or concurrently)
- ► Non-Hodgkin lymphoma of the breast is usually secondary to disseminated disease
- ► Considered primary breast lymphoma when isolated to the breast
- ► Typically presents as a palpable mass
  - ▪ 30% to 40% have associated axillary adenopathy
- ► May appear as circumscribed mass (as in this case) or ill-defined, obscured mass on mammogram
  - ▪ Spiculated margins uncommon
  - ▪ Infrequently may present with multiple masses
  - ▪ No associated calcifications
- ► Ultrasound appearance varies
  - ▪ Hypoechoic to nearly anechoic mass
  - ▪ Posterior acoustic enhancement common
    - ◆ Take care to avoid misinterpreting as a cyst

Management

- ► Ultrasound-guided core needle biopsy for tissue diagnosis
- ► When biopsy reveals lymphoma, staging recommended to exclude systemic disease

Selected References/Further Reading

Cardenosa G. *Clinical Breast Imaging: A Patient-Focused Teaching File*. Philadelphia: Lippincott Williams & Wilkins, 2007:366-367.

Liberman L, et al. Non-Hodgkin's lymphoma of the breast: imaging characteristics and correlation with histopathologic findings. *Radiology* 1994;192:157-160.

Zack JR, et al. Primary breast lymphoma originating in a benign intramammary lymph node. *AJR* 2001;177:177-178.

History

► Asymptomatic woman with a personal history of left breast cancer. The patient underwent breast conservation therapy (BCT) one year ago. This is her first post-treatment diagnostic mammogram

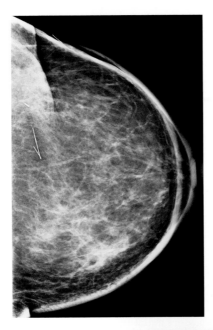
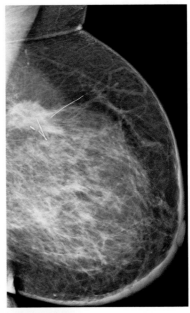

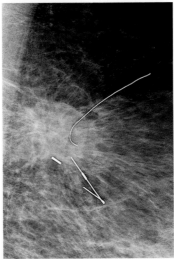

Case 42 Retained Localization Wire

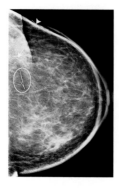 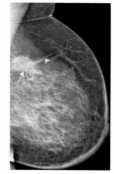 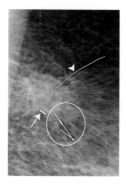

Findings

▶ Expected changes of lumpectomy and radiation therapy are present
  (architectural distortion at the lumpectomy site, trabecular thickening, skin
  thickening and edema)
  ▪ A portion of a localizing wire, including the distal "hook," is present adjacent
    to the lumpectomy bed (*circle*)
  ▪ A surgical clip is present (*arrow*)
  ▪ A scar marker was placed on the skin (*arrowhead*)

Differential Diagnosis

▶ None—classic appearance demonstrated

Teaching Points

▶ Wire localization is frequently performed in advance of surgical excision
  ▪ Useful for non-palpable masses
  ▪ Decreases the rate of positive margins when performed in conjunction with
    specimen radiography
▶ Wire may be inadvertently transected during surgery
▶ Retained wires are uncommon
  ▪ Usually asymptomatic
  ▪ Complications are rare, but migration of wire fragments has been reported
    ◆ If partially contained in pectoralis muscle, complications more likely

Management

▶ Specimen radiography should be performed following all preoperative wire
  localizations to evaluate inclusion of the target and to confirm complete removal
  of the wire
  ▪ If the wire is not entirely included in the specimen, the surgeon should be
    alerted immediately in the operating room to facilitate prompt removal
▶ The patient should be informed if a retained wire fragment is present
  ▪ Consider short-term follow-up to assess for migration
  ▪ Offer re-excision

Selected References/Further Reading

Ikeda DM. *Breast Imaging: The Requisites*. Philadelphia: Elsevier Mosby, 2004:315.
Kopans DB. Migration of breast biopsy localizing wire [letter]. *AJR* 1988;151:614-615.
Motrey JS, et al. Wire fragments after needle localization. *AJR* 1996;167:1267-1269.

History

▶ 45-year-old woman with a new, soft, palpable mass in the right breast. A metallic BB marks the area of concern

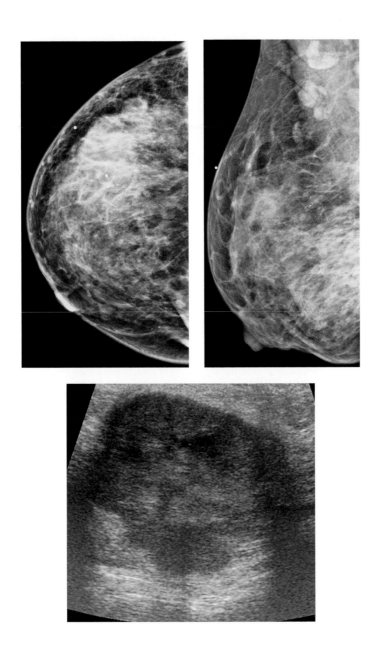

Case 43 Medullary Carcinoma

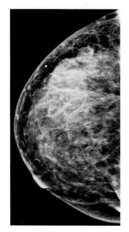 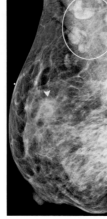 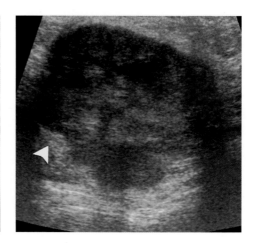

Findings

- ▶ Mammogram
  - ▪ Equal-density, non-calcified mass that is predominantly obscured by surrounding dense glandular tissue (difficult to discern on the CC view). There is a partially circumscribed margin superiorly on the MLO view (*arrowhead*)
  - ▪ Prominent axillary lymph nodes are present (*circle*)
- ▶ Ultrasound
  - ▪ Heterogeneously hypoechoic irregular mass with posterior acoustic enhancement
  - ▪ Note that the superficial margin is smooth and circumscribed, while the posterior margin is microlobulated, with the suggestion of an echogenic halo (*arrowhead*)

Differential Diagnosis

- ▶ Invasive ductal carcinoma (high-grade)
- ▶ Mucinous carcinoma
- ▶ Phyllodes tumor

Teaching Points

- ▶ Variant of invasive ductal carcinoma
  - ▪ Less than 5% of breast cancers
  - ▪ Typical and atypical subtypes exist
- ▶ More common in
  - ▪ Younger patients
  - ▪ Patients with Japanese or African-American heritage
- ▶ May mimic a benign mass on imaging and clinical exam
- ▶ Mammographic appearance
  - ▪ Round or oval
  - ▪ Equal-density or high-density
  - ▪ Margins may be partially circumscribed
    - ◆ Spiculated margins atypical

- Calcifications uncommon
  - Axillary adenopathy common but may be reactive rather than metastatic disease
- ▶ Ultrasound appearance
  - Round
  - Hypoechoic, or nearly anechoic with posterior acoustic enhancement
  - Most margins appear circumscribed, but usually a portion is irregular or angular
  - Internal vascular flow with color Doppler

Management

- ▶ Ultrasound-guided core needle biopsy for tissue diagnosis
- ▶ Typical variety has better prognosis than invasive ductal carcinoma, with a 5-year survival of 89% to 95%

Selected References/Further Reading

Bassett LW, et al. *Diagnosis of Diseases of the Breast*, 2nd ed. Philadelphia: WB Saunders Co., 2005:501-504.
Majid AS, de Paredes ES, et al. Missed breast carcinoma: pitfalls and pearls. *RadioGraphics* 2003;23:881-895.
Stavros AT. *Breast Ultrasound*. Philadelphia: Lippincott Williams & Wilkins, 2004:641-645.

History

▶ 47-year-old woman with a palpable mass in the left axilla

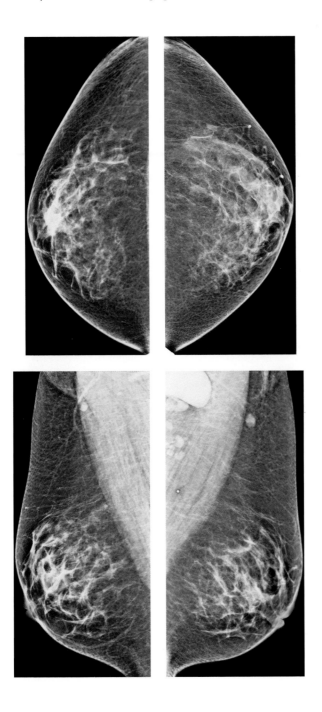

Case 44 Mammographically Occult Breast Cancer Presenting with Metastatic Axillary Lymphadenopathy

Findings
- ▶ Enlarged, dense, axillary lymph nodes
- ▶ No mammographically detectable mass, calcifications, architectural distortion, or other sign of malignancy

Differential Diagnosis
- ▶ Lymphoma
- ▶ Metastatic carcinoma from extra-mammary site
- ▶ Reactive adenopathy
  - ▪ Systemic illness
  - ▪ Cat-scratch disease

Teaching Points
- ▶ Uncommon presentation of breast carcinoma

Management
- ▶ Ultrasound-guided fine-needle aspiration of the lymph node for diagnosis
  - ▪ Core needle biopsy may be requested to identify tumor receptor status in patients undergoing neoadjuvant chemotherapy
- ▶ When diagnosis of metastatic adenocarcinoma consistent with a breast primary is confirmed, careful mammographic evaluation is warranted
  - ▪ High-quality imaging is imperative in these patients
- ▶ Contrast-enhanced breast MR should be performed if mammography is negative
  - ▪ Lesions detected are typically small and/or multifocal
  - ▪ MR-guided biopsy may identify the "occult" malignancy
- ▶ Treatment is controversial
  - ▪ Mastectomy has historically been the treatment of choice, and is still an accepted treatment option
    - ◆ Primary tumor not always found in the mastectomy specimen
  - ▪ Recently, whole breast radiation without mastectomy has been utilized when the primary malignancy is not detected

Selected References/Further Reading

Ikeda DM. *Breast Imaging: The Requisites*. Elsevier Mosby, 2004, 304-305.
Morris EA, et al. MR imaging of the breast in patients with occult primary breast carcinoma. *Radiology* 1997;205:437-440.

History

▶ 57 year-old woman with spontaneous left bloody nipple discharge referred for galactography (ductogram)

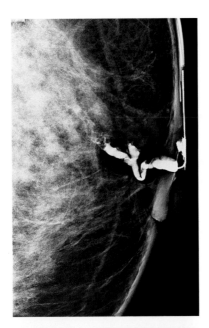

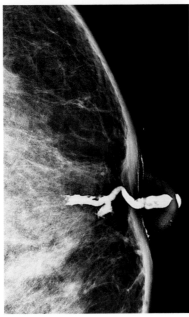

Case 45 Papilloma (Appearance on Galactogram)

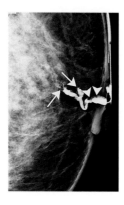 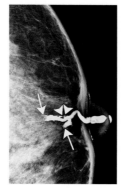

Findings

▶ There are multiple intraductal masses seen as multiple filling defects (*arrowheads*) and as abrupt termination of the contrast filled ducts (*arrows*)

Differential Diagnosis

▶ Ductal carcinoma in situ (DCIS)
▶ Papillary carcinoma
▶ Papillomatosis/multiple papillomas

Teaching Points

▶ Papillomas are benign ductal neoplasms
  ▪ May bleed into the duct, causing nipple discharge
  ▪ Most common cause of bloody nipple discharge
▶ Pathologic discharge is usually defined as persistent, unilateral, serous or bloody, spontaneous secretion from a single duct
  ▪ Benign bloody discharge may occur in late pregnancy, early postpartum
▶ Diagnostic mammography is the first-line imaging evaluation of pathologic nipple discharge
  ▪ Assess for suspicious calcifications or masses
▶ Galactography (ductography) is reserved for the evaluation of pathologic nipple discharge
  ▪ Direct injection of contrast into the discharging duct
  ▪ Technique:
    ◆ Typically performed immediately prior to surgical excision
    ◆ Magnifying glass and high-intensity lamp help with visualization of the duct opening
    ◆ 27- or 30-gauge straight or curved needle-catheter system is used to cannulate the discharging duct
    ◆ Water-soluble contrast (e.g., Conray 60)
      • Eliminate air bubbles in tubing
      • Include a few drops of methylene blue if requested by surgeon for same-day surgical excision
      • Inject 0.2 to 0.3 cc slowly

- ◆ Magnification CC and ML images after injection
- ◆ If extravasation occurs, must reschedule patient in 7 to 10 days
- ▪ Contraindications
  - ◆ Contrast allergy
  - ◆ Prior nipple/areolar surgery
- ▶ As breast surgeons increasingly perform ductoscopy and/or ductal lavage to evaluate pathologic nipple discharge, galactography is less commonly requested

Management

- ▶ Directed duct excision (microductectomy) is both diagnostic and therapeutic for resolving bloody nipple discharge

Selected References/Further Reading

Bassett LW, et al. *Diagnosis of Diseases of the Breast*, 2nd ed. Philadelphia: WB Saunders Co., 2005:430-432.
Cardenosa G, et al. Ductography of the breast: technique and findings. *AJR* 1994;162:1082-1087.
Slawson SH, et al. Ductography: how to and what if? *RadioGraphics* 2001;21:133-150.

History

▶ Screening mammogram

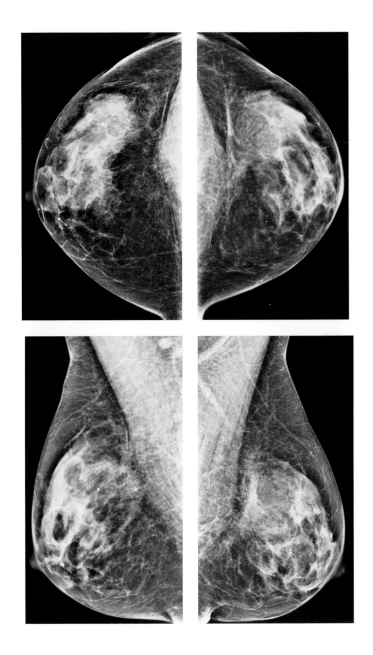

Case 46   Explantation (Removal) of Bilateral Subglandular Implants

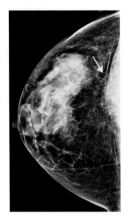 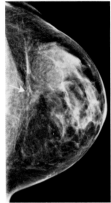 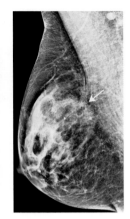 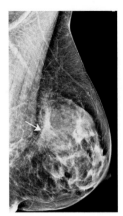

Findings

► Architectural distortion seen on both the CC and MLO views in the posterior breasts (retroglandular fat) centrally (*arrows*)

Differential Diagnosis

► None—classic appearance demonstrated

Teaching Points

► Clinical history is important in interpretation of imaging studies
► Imaging findings after implant removal (explantation) are variable
  ▪ May appear normal
  ▪ Fat necrosis/dystrophic calcifications are common
  ▪ Capsular calcifications, dense scarring, architectural distortion and/or residual free silicone may result in a more suspicious appearance
  ▪ Fluid may accumulate in the implant cavity (seroma)

Management

► BI-RADS® Category 2: Benign findings
► Annual screening mammography

Selected References/Further Reading

Cardenosa, G. *Clinical Breast Imaging: A Patient-Focused Teaching File*. Philadelphia: Lippincott Williams & Wilkins, 2007:168-169.
Ikeda DM. *Breast Imaging: The Requisites*. Philadelphia: Elsevier Mosby, 2004:264.
Middleton MS, McNamara MP. *Breast Implant Imaging*. Philadelphia: Lippincott Williams & Wilkins, 2003.

History

► Screening mammogram (right breast images shown)

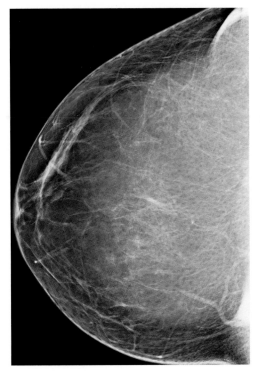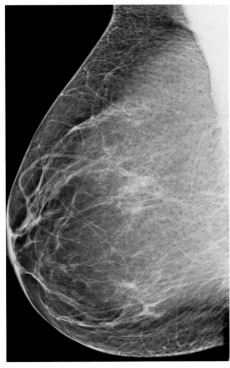

Case 47 Sternalis Muscle

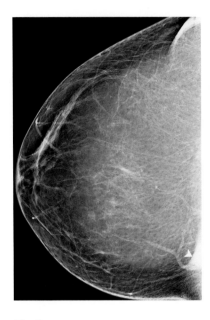
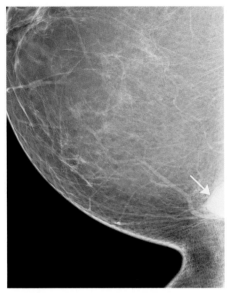

Findings

- ▶ Triangular or "sail-shaped" density in the medial breast on the CC view (*arrowhead*); no correlate is present on the MLO view
  - ▪ Cleavage view demonstrates the finding to greatest advantage (*arrow*)

Differential Diagnosis

- ▶ None—classic appearance demonstrated

Teaching Points

- ▶ Normal variant of chest wall musculature
  - ▪ Muscle oriented parallel to sternum
  - ▪ No known function
- ▶ Uncommon, less than 8% of the population
  - ▪ Occasionally seen on CC view of mammogram
- ▶ Typically triangular, flame- or "sail-shaped," but may appear rounded
- ▶ If the appearance is not classic, recall the patient for a diagnostic evaluation in order to exclude a true mass

Management

- ▶ Annual screening mammography

Selected References/Further Reading

Bassett LW, et al. *Diagnosis of Diseases of the Breast*, 2nd ed. Philadelphia: WB Saunders Co., 2005:393-395.
Bradley FM, et al. The sternalis muscle: An unusual normal finding seen on mammography. *AJR* 1996;166:33-36.
Ikeda DM. *Breast Imaging: The Requisites*. Philadelphia: Elsevier Mosby, 2004:26-27.

History

▶ Abnormal screening mammogram. Diagnostic mammogram and ultrasound images shown

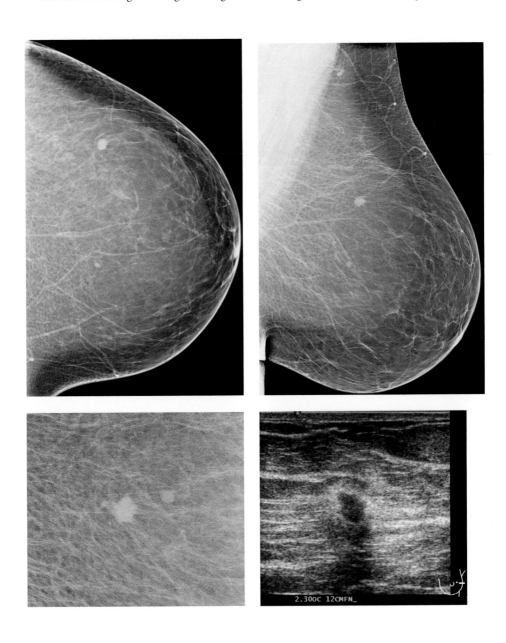

Case 48 Tubular Carcinoma

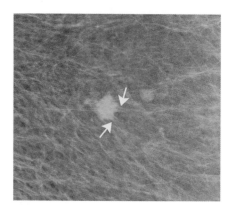 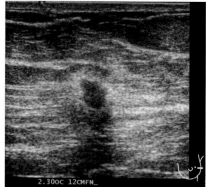

Findings

- ▶ Mammogram
  - ▪ Small, high-density, irregular mass with spiculated margins
  - ▪ Note the spicules extending into surrounding fatty tissue on the spot magnification view (*arrows*)
- ▶ Ultrasound
  - ▪ Irregular, hypoechoic, non-parallel (vertical orientation) mass with posterior acoustic shadowing and a subtle echogenic rim

Differential Diagnosis

- ▶ Invasive ductal carcinoma
- ▶ Radial scar (classically has long spiculations with central lucency)
  - ▪ Tubular cancer may coexist with radial scar/radial sclerosing lesions (RS/RSL)
- ▶ Invasive lobular carcinoma

Teaching Points

- ▶ Special type of well-differentiated invasive ductal carcinoma
  - ▪ Uncommon, accounts for less than 5% of all invasive breast carcinomas
  - ▪ Named for histologic appearance: tubule formation with surrounding desmoplastic reaction
- ▶ Usually screen detected
- ▶ Classic imaging features demonstrated in this case
  - ▪ Slow-growing (small when detected) and may appear stable mammographically for years
  - ▪ May have associated calcifications
- ▶ Favorable prognosis, typically without metastasis at diagnosis

Management

- ▶ Ultrasound-guided core biopsy for tissue diagnosis
- ▶ Opinions vary regarding the association between RS/RSL and tubular carcinoma
  - ▪ When RS/RSL is found at core needle biopsy, *and* suspicious imaging features are present mammographically (architectural distortion/spiculated mass), surgical excision is recommended to exclude coexisting malignancy
    - ◆ Data evolving

Selected References/Further Reading

Bassett LW, et al. *Diagnosis of Diseases of the Breast*, 2nd ed. Philadelphia: WB Saunders Co., 2005:506-508.

Javid CH, et al. Tubular carcinoma of the breast: results of a large contemporary series. *Am J Surg* 2009; 197:674-677.

Stavros AT. *Breast Ultrasound*. Philadelphia: Lippincott Williams & Wilkins, 2004:703-709.

History

▶ 64-year-old woman with a personal history of breast cancer, for which the patient was treated with right mastectomy 2 years ago. She reports a new palpable mass adjacent to the mastectomy scar

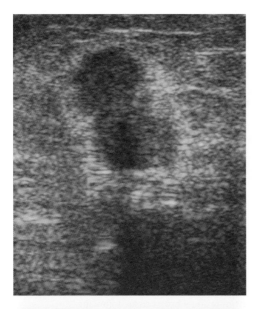

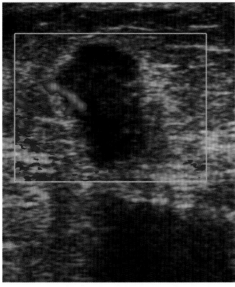

Case 49   Recurrent Breast Cancer after Mastectomy

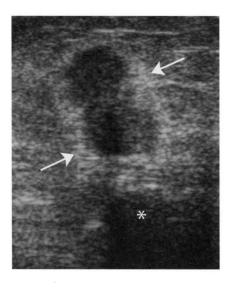

Findings

► Irregular, hypoechoic, solid mass with a hyperechoic rim (*arrows*) and non-parallel (vertical) orientation. An underlying rib limits evaluation of the posterior acoustic features (*asterisk*)

Differential Diagnosis

► New primary breast malignancy arising from residual breast tissue following mastectomy
► Postoperative fibrosis (unlikely in this case given imaging features)

Teaching Points

► Mastectomy significantly reduces the risk of local recurrence but does not eliminate risk entirely
  ▪ Recurrence is most likely to occur in the chest wall or in skin
  ▪ Typically detected with clinical exam
    ◆ 60% to 80% occur within 2 years of mastectomy
► Ultrasound is the first-line imaging modality when patients present with clinical symptoms at the mastectomy site
► Typically, recurrence manifests as an irregular, hypoechoic solid mass (similar to a primary breast malignancy)
► Mammography has a limited role in patients post mastectomy
  ▪ Surveillance of mastectomy sites with annual mammography is controversial and not routinely performed at most institutions
  ▪ Diagnostic mammography may be performed in symptomatic patients but is rarely contributory
► Palpable masses in reconstructed myocutaneous flaps (e.g., TRAM) most commonly represent fat necrosis and not recurrence
  ▪ Mammography will usually confirm the diagnosis and obviate the need for ultrasound or biopsy

- Four types of mastectomies
  - Radical (includes resection of the pectoralis muscle, overlying skin, and axillary lymph node dissection; rarely performed today)
  - Modified radical
  - Simple
  - Skin-sparing (more options for reconstruction)

Management

- Ultrasound-guided core needle biopsy for tissue diagnosis
  - If there is scant tissue surrounding the mass ultrasound-guided fine needle aspiration (FNA) may be preferable and more technically feasible

Selected References/Further Reading

Bland K, Copeland E. *The Breast: Comprehensive Management of Benign and Malignant Disorders*. St. Louis, MO: Saunders, 2004: Chapters 39 and 76.

Kim SM, Park JM. Normal and abnormal ultrasound findings at the mastectomy site. *RadioGraphics* 2004;24:357-365.

Stavros AT. *Breast Ultrasound*. Philadelphia: Lippincott Williams & Wilkins, 2004:803, 814.

History

▶ Screening mammogram

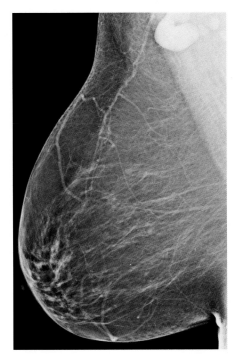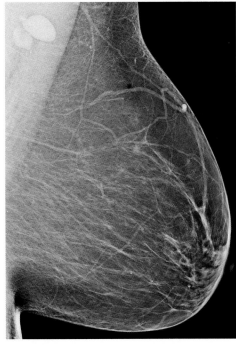

Case 50 Bilateral Axillary Adenopathy Secondary to HIV Infection

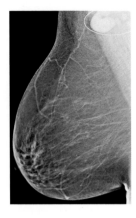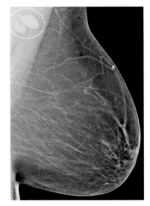

Findings

▶ Multiple, bilateral, enlarged axillary lymph nodes (*circles*) *without* associated calcifications. No suspicious finding is present in the breast parenchyma

Differential Diagnosis

▶ Bilateral axillary adenopathy
- Lymphoma
- Collagen vascular disease/rheumatoid arthritis
- Granulomatous disease (sarcoidosis, tuberculosis)
- Metastatic disease

Teaching Points

▶ Lymph nodes are frequently included on MLO projections
▶ Differential considerations differ if unilateral versus bilateral adenopathy
▶ Ultrasound may help characterize and narrow differential
- Eccentric cortical thickening suggests metastatic disease
  - ◆ Loss of fatty hilum is highly suspicious
- Uniform, smooth cortical thickening suggests reactive adenopathy
- "Snowstorm" appearance is consistent with silicone adenopathy

Management

▶ Correlate with clinical history
▶ If no known history to explain findings, further evaluation with ultrasound and biopsy of lymph nodes for diagnosis should be considered
- Ultrasound-guided fine-needle aspiration or core needle biopsy

Selected References/Further Reading

American College of Radiology (ACR). ACR BI-RADS®—Mammography, 4th ed. *ACR Breast Imaging Reporting and Data Systems, Breast Imaging Atlas*. Reston, VA: American College of Radiology, 2003:172-173.

Bassett LW, et al. *Diagnosis of Diseases of the Breast*, 2nd ed. Philadelphia: WB Saunders Co., 2005:407-413.

Walsh R, et al. Axillary lymph nodes: mammographic, pathologic and clinical correlation. *AJR* 1997;168:33-38.

History

▶ Screening mammogram

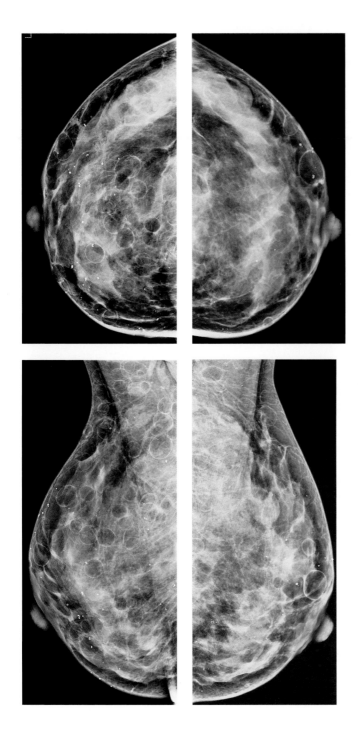

Case 51 Steatocystoma Multiplex

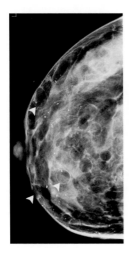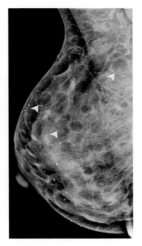

Findings

▶ Innumerable, fat-density, circumscribed, round masses with thin capsules, distributed bilaterally (*arrowheads*)
  ▪ May be more numerous in the axillary tail

Differential Diagnosis

▶ None—classic appearance demonstrated
  ▪ May project over the breast parenchyma on mammographic views

Teaching Points

▶ Steatocystomas are small, intradermal, 1 to 20-mm papules containing oily fluid (hence fat density on mammography)
  ▪ Benign lesions
  ▪ Appear in adolescence
  ▪ Distributed over the trunk, back, proximal extremities, and external genitalia
▶ Intradermal location distinguishes them from breast parenchymal oil cysts/fat necrosis
▶ Tangent (horizontal beam) film may show fat–fluid meniscus
▶ Uncommon disorder
  ▪ Autosomal dominant inheritance pattern described, but many cases are sporadic

Management

▶ Annual screening mammography

Selected References/Further Reading

Bassett LW, et al. *Diagnosis of Diseases of the Breast*, 2nd ed. Philadelphia: WB Saunders Co., 2005:401-402.

Pollack AH, Kuerer HM. Steatocystoma multiplex: appearance at mammography. *Radiology* 1991;180:836-838.

History

▶ 40-year-old woman with a palpable mass in the left breast. Additional history withheld

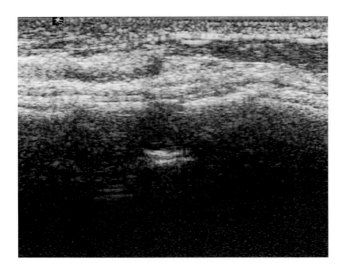

Case 52 Saline Implant Valve (Presenting as a Palpable Mass)

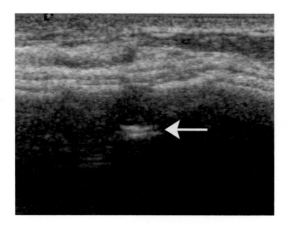 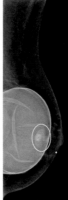

Findings

- ▶ Ultrasound
  - ▪ Characteristic appearance of the filling valve within saline breast implants. Note the hyperechoic linear structure deep to the envelope (*arrow*)
- ▶ Mammogram
  - ▪ The metallic BB denoting the patient's area of concern projects over the saline implant valve. The filling valve is easily seen mammographically (*circle*)

Differential Diagnosis

- ▶ None—classic appearance demonstrated

Teaching Points

- ▶ Inflatable saline implants, tissue expanders, and some double-lumen implants have filling valves or ports
  - ▪ Instilled with sterile saline at the time of implantation
  - ▪ Allows adjustment of size
  - ▪ Different valve types
    - ◆ Leaflet
      - • Unlikely to present as palpable mass
    - ◆ Diaphragm
      - • More common
- ▶ Valves usually placed in subareolar tissue
  - ▪ May migrate as implant rotates
  - ▪ May evert and become palpable (normally the valve protrudes inward)
- ▶ Patients may present with mobile "mass"

Management

- ▶ Reassure patient
- ▶ Annual screening mammography

Selected References/Further Reading

Middleton MS, McNamara MP. *Breast Implant Imaging*. Philadelphia: Lippincott Williams & Wilkins, 2003.

Stavros AT. *Breast Ultrasound*. Philadelphia: Lippincott Williams & Wilkins, 2004:219-221.

History

▶ 46-year-old woman with a palpable thickening in her left breast

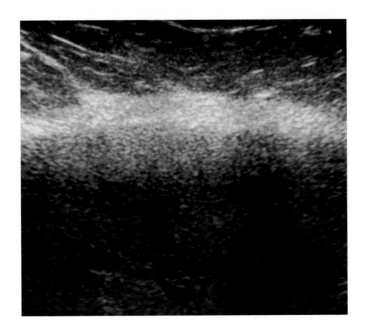

Case 53 Ultrasound Appearance of Extracapsular Rupture of a Silicone Implant

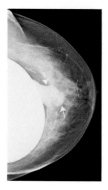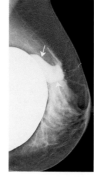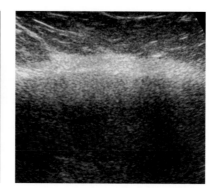

Findings

- ► Ultrasound
  - ▪ "Snowstorm" or "dirty shadowing" appearance of free silicone (increased echogenicity in the near-field with loss of posterior detail)
- ► Mammogram
  - ▪ Confirms that the lobular density extends anterior from the implant (*arrows*), and is consistent with leaking silicone

Differential Diagnosis

- ► None—classic appearance demonstrated

Teaching Points

- ► Extracapsular rupture is silicone gel that has leaked into the soft tissue outside both the implant membrane (shell) and the fibrous capsule
  - ▪ Fibrous capsule develops shortly after implantation
- ► Silicone causes reverberation and refraction of ultrasound waves, resulting in "snowstorm" or "dirty-shadowing" appearance
  - ▪ Appearance is pathognomonic
  - ▪ Difficult to evaluate deeper tissue
- ► Silicone implant rupture is typically asymptomatic
- ► Over time, most implants will fail (rupture)
- ► There is no proven increased risk for breast cancer or collagen vascular disease in patients with ruptured silicone implants

Management

- ► Inform patient of extracapsular implant rupture
  - ▪ Patient may consider explantation or revision
    - ◆ Difficult to remove all free silicone in most cases
- ► Annual screening mammography

Selected References/Further Reading

Bassett LW, et al. *Diagnosis of Diseases of the Breast*, 2nd ed. Philadelphia: WB Saunders Co., 2005: Chapter 32.

Middleton MS, McNamara MP. *Breast Implant Imaging.* Philadelphia: Lippincott Williams & Wilkins, 2003.

History

▶ 56-year-old asymptomatic woman presents for her annual screening mammogram (CC views shown)

Three years ago

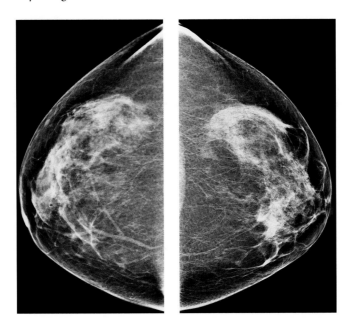

Current exam

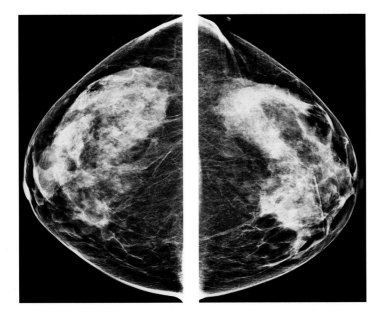

Case 54 Effects of Hormone Replacement Therapy (HRT)

Findings

- ► Exams performed 3 years apart demonstrate interval increase of glandular tissue in a bilateral and symmetric pattern. There is no suspicious finding in either breast

Differential Diagnosis

- ► Interval weight loss (which results in increased compressibility of breast tissue)
- ► Lactational change (in a lactating patient)

Teaching Points

- ► Breast parenchyma normally involutes in postmenopausal patients
  - ▪ Mammographic density usually diminishes
- ► Developing densities may occur in postmenopausal patients on HRT
  - ▪ May be symmetric and global (as in this case)
    - ◆ Variable time frame (months to years) for developing after HRT started
  - ▪ May be focal
    - ◆ View with suspicion to exclude malignancy
    - ◆ Diagnostic mammogram and ultrasound
- ► Natural involution resumes when HRT is discontinued in most patients
- ► Breast parenchymal density is considered an independent risk factor for development of breast cancer
- ► The Women's Health Initiative (2002) demonstrated increased risk of invasive breast cancer for women on combination HRT (estrogen and progesterone)

Management

- ► Correlate with the clinical history
- ► If bilateral and symmetric, annual screening mammography is appropriate
- ► If there is a new focal asymmetry, diagnostic mammogram and ultrasound are required to exclude a developing malignancy

Selected References/Further Reading

Berg W, et al. *Diagnostic Imaging of the Breast*. Salt Lake City, UT: Amirsys Inc., 2006: Part IV, Chapter 5, 2-5.

Roussouw JE, et al. Risks and benefits of estrogen plus progestin in healthy postmenopausal women: Principal results from the Women's Health Initiative randomized controlled trial. *JAMA* 2002;288:321-333.

Rutter CM, et al. Changes in breast density associated with initiation, discontinuation, and continuing use of hormone replacement therapy. *JAMA* 2001;285:171-176.

History

▸ 43-year-old woman with a firm palpable mass in the right upper outer quadrant. A metallic BB denotes the area of palpable concern

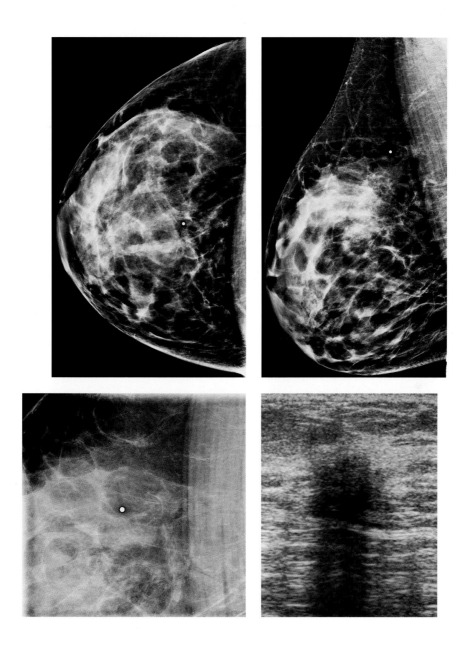

Case 55   Granular Cell Tumor (GCT)

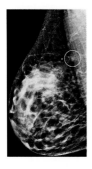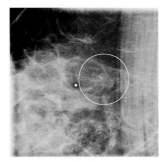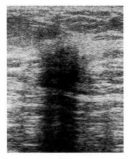

Findings

▶ Mammogram
  ▪ Subtle, equal-density, irregular mass with spiculated margins (*circles*)
▶ Ultrasound
  ▪ Irregular, hypoechoic mass with microlobulated margins and dense posterior acoustic shadowing

Differential Diagnosis

▶ Invasive ductal carcinoma (IDC)
▶ Invasive lobular carcinoma (ILC)
▶ Tubular carcinoma

Teaching Points

▶ Rare
▶ Typically benign, but can be locally aggressive or malignant (2%)
  ▪ 5% to 10% are multiple
  ▪ When deep may adhere to pectoralis fascia
▶ Mimics invasive ductal carcinoma (IDC) both radiographically and pathologically
  ▪ IDC is far more common
  ▪ Misdiagnosis possible
▶ Axillary adenopathy is atypical
▶ Can occur anywhere in the body
  ▪ Head and neck most common
  ▪ 5% of all GCTs occur in breast
▶ Probably arise from Schwann cells in lobular breast stroma

Management

▶ BI-RADS® Category 5: Highly suspicious for malignancy
▶ Ultrasound-guided core needle biopsy for tissue diagnosis
▶ Good prognosis
  ▪ Wide local excision recommended when diagnosis confirmed at core needle biopsy

Selected References/Further Reading

Brown AC, et al. Granular cell tumour of the breast. *Surg Oncol* 2010; Epub Jan. 12.
Yang WT, et al. Sonographic and mammographic appearances of granular cell tumors of the breast with pathological correlation. *J Clin Ultrasound* 2006;34:153-160.

History

► Abnormal screening mammogram. Spot magnification mediolateral (90 degree) image from diagnostic evaluation shown

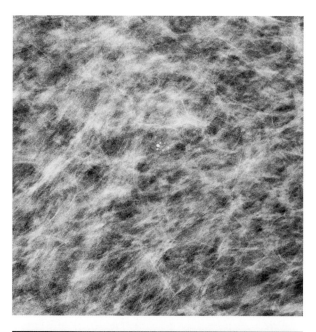

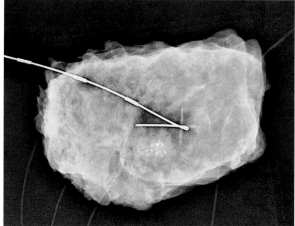

Case 56   Lobular Carcinoma In Situ (LCIS)

Findings

► Mammogram
  ▪ Solitary cluster of predominantly round calcifications. No associated mass or architectural distortion
► Specimen radiograph demonstrates inclusion of the calcifications at excision

Differential Diagnosis

► Ductal carcinoma in situ (DCIS)
► Atypical lobular hyperplasia (ALH)
► Benign calcifications (e.g., fibrocystic change, sclerosing adenosis)

Teaching Points

► "Lobular neoplasia" includes LCIS and ALH
  ▪ High-risk lesions associated with increased risk of breast cancer bilaterally
    ◆ Often multifocal and bilateral
  ▪ Relative risk approximately 10x
► Associated with invasive lobular carcinoma (ILC)
► High-risk lesions diagnosed at core needle biopsy may represent malignancy when surgically excised
  ▪ Variable reports of "upstage" to malignancy (10-27%)
► Usually mammographically occult or nonspecific in appearance
  ▪ Found incidentally at core needle biopsy
    ◆ Usually when biopsy performed for suspicious calcifications
► More frequent in white patients than African-American patients
► Mean age 45 years

Management

► Excisional biopsy is recommended when LCIS or ALH are present in a core needle biopsy (CNB) specimen
► While LCIS and ALH found at CNB require surgical excision, re-excision is not required when present at the margins of a surgical specimen
► High-risk surveillance pattern may be recommended
  ▪ Annual MR for additional screening
► Chemoprevention used in some patients (e.g., tamoxifen)
► Rarely, patients may elect prophylactic mastectomies particularly if other risk factors are present

Selected References/Further Reading

Berg WA. Imaging-guided breast biopsy and management of high-risk lesions. *Radiol Clin North Am* 2004;42:935-946.

Berg WA, et al. Atypical lobular hyperplasia or lobular carcinoma in situ at core-needle breast biopsy. *Radiology* 2001;218:503-509.

Foster MC, et al. Lobular carcinoma in situ or atypical lobular hyperplasia at core needle biopsy: Is excisional biopsy necessary? *Radiology* 231; 813-819, 2004.

History

▶ Abnormal screening mammogram. Spot magnification CC and ML images from diagnostic evaluation shown

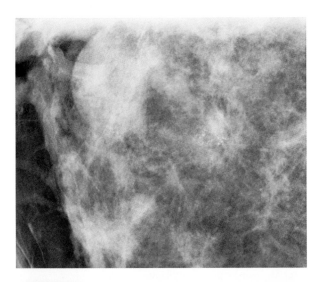

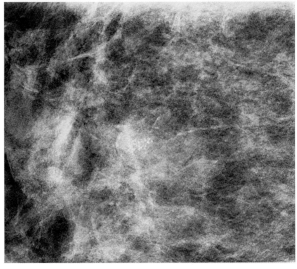

Case 57 Low-grade Ductal Carcinoma In Situ

Findings

▸ Solitary cluster of amorphous microcalcifications

Differential Diagnosis

▸ Atypical ductal hyperplasia (ADH)
▸ Benign calcifications (e.g., fibrocystic change, sclerosing adenosis)
▸ Lobular neoplasia (LCIS, ALH)

Teaching Points

▸ Non-invasive (Stage 0) carcinoma
  ▪ Potential to become invasive
▸ DCIS is graded as low, intermediate, high
  ▪ Low grade refers to low nuclear grade (low mitotic activity)
    ◆ No necrosis
  ▪ Little prognostic value
▸ Classically clustered, amorphous/indistinct microcalcifications on screening mammography
  ▪ Also described as "powdery" or "cotton-ball like"
  ▪ "Amorphous" is preferred terminology in BI-RADS® lexicon
▸ Located within the terminal duct lobular unit (TDLU)
▸ May be mammographically stable for years; however, stability of microcalcifications should never dissuade biopsy of suspicious findings
▸ Rarely low-grade DCIS may be associated with a mass that is detected on clinical exam or by imaging

Management

▸ Stereotactic core needle biopsy for tissue diagnosis
  ▪ Calcifications must be present in core tissue submitted for pathologic analysis
▸ To assist in surgical planning, document the extent of disease
  ▪ Biopsy of additional microcalcifications may be required
  ▪ Most patients will be candidates for breast conserving therapy
  ▪ Mastectomy may be required if extensive
▸ Patients with estrogen-receptor–positive DCIS are typically offered tamoxifen

Selected References/Further Reading

American College of Radiology (ACR). ACR BI-RADS®—Mammography, 4th Ed. *ACR Breast Imaging Reporting and Data Systems, Breast Imaging Atlas.* Reston, VA: American College of Radiology, 2003:92-97.

Bassett LW, et al. *Diagnosis of Diseases of the Breast*, 2nd ed. Philadelphia: WB Saunders Co., 2005: Chapter 26.

Silverstein MJ. *Ductal Carcinoma In Situ of the Breast*, 2nd ed. Philadelphia: Lippincott Williams & Wilkins, 2002: Chapter 10.

Tot T, Tabar L, Dean P. *Practical Breast Pathology*. New York: Thieme, 2005: Chapter 4.

History

▶ 43-year-old diabetic woman (type 1, diagnosed in childhood) with a firm, palpable mass in the left breast. A metallic BB marks the area of palpable concern

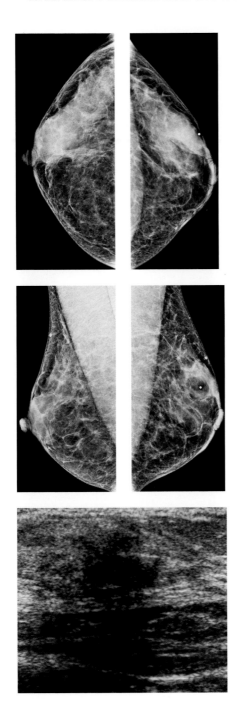

Case 58   Diabetic Mastopathy

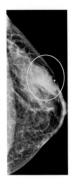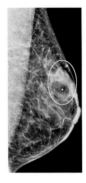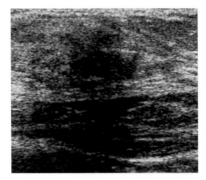

Findings

▶ Mammogram
  ▪ There is a vague increased density without a discrete mass or architectural distortion (*circles*) in the area of palpable concern. No suspicious calcifications are present
▶ Ultrasound
  ▪ There is focal posterior acoustic shadowing with the suggestion of an indistinct mass

Differential Diagnosis

▶ Invasive ductal carcinoma (IDC)
▶ Invasive lobular carcinoma (ILC)
▶ Stromal fibrosis

Teaching Points

▶ Rare
▶ Also known as diabetic fibrous breast disease
▶ Classically patients present with firm, palpable mass(es)
  ▪ Occurs in type 1 diabetics of long duration (average 20 years)
▶ Mammogram appearance: symmetric density without a discrete mass
▶ Ultrasound appearance: ill-defined mass, frequently with posterior acoustic shadowing
▶ No increased risk for breast cancer
▶ MR not helpful in discriminating the diagnosis

Management

▶ Imaging is nonspecific; therefore, tissue diagnosis with ultrasound-guided core needle biopsy is recommended
  ▪ Fine-needle aspiration does not provide sufficient tissue to establish the diagnosis
  ▪ Some patients may require excisional biopsy to achieve concordant results

Selected References/Further Reading

Bassett LW, et al. *Diagnosis of Diseases of the Breast*, 2nd ed. Philadelphia: WB Saunders Co., 2005:442-443.

Thorncroft K, et al. The diagnosis and management of diabetic mastopathy. *Breast J* 2007;13:607-613.

History

▶ Screening mammogram

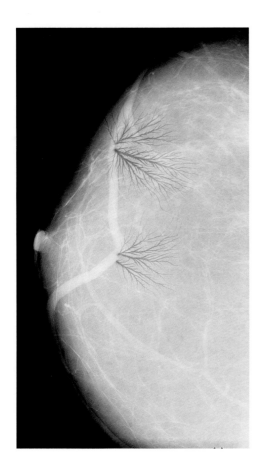

Case 59   Static Artifact on Analog (Film-screen) Mammogram

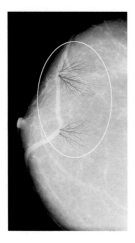

Findings

▶ Star-burst, non-anatomic "plus-density" (darker) artifact resulting from static electric discharge at film surface prior to processing (*circle*)

Differential Diagnosis

▶ None—classic appearance demonstrated

Teaching Points

▶ Analog (film-screen) mammography is susceptible to artifacts
  ▪ May obscure normal and/or abnormal findings
  ▪ May mimic suspicious findings (e.g., calcifications)
▶ Artifacts may arise from film manufacturing or handling, equipment-related problems, processing, environmental issues, or positioning problems
  ▪ Processing is the primary source of artifacts for analog imaging
▶ Static marks may appear when air in the darkroom is too dry
  ▪ Humidity should be between 30% and 50%
▶ Digital mammography is also subject to artifacts (but not covered here)

Management

▶ Annual screening mammography
▶ Review quality control of imaging in accordance with MQSA guidelines/regulations
  ▪ Consult lead quality control (QC) tech
  ▪ Consult physicist
▶ Refer to FDA website *www.fda.gov/cdrh/mammography*

Selected References/Further Reading

Andolina VF, et al. *Mammographic Imaging: A Practical Guide,* 2nd ed. Philadelphia: Lippincott Williams & Wilkins, 2001: Chapter 6.

Bassett LW, et al. *Diagnosis of Diseases of the Breast*, 2nd ed. Philadelphia: WB Saunders Co., 2005:82-84.

Hendrick RE, et al. *ACT Mammography Quality Control Manual*, 4th ed. American College of Radiology, 1999.

History

▶ Abnormal screening mammogram. Images from diagnostic evaluation shown

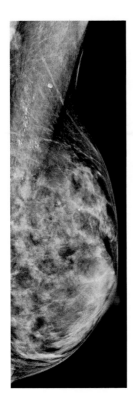
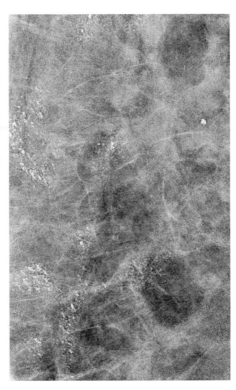

Case 60 Tattoo Artifact

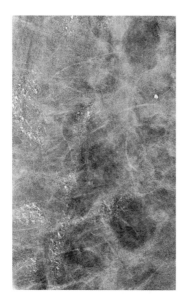 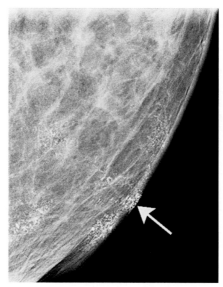

Findings

▶ Multiple groups of heterogeneous hyperdensities. Tangent view confirms that they reside in the dermis (*arrow*). Clinical exam confirmed a tattoo in this location

Differential Diagnosis

▶ Parenchymal microcalcifications

Teaching Points

▶ Multiple materials applied to skin contain radiodense material and may mimic suspicious microcalcifications
  ▪ Antiperspirant containing aluminum most common
  ▪ Cream, ointment, powder
▶ Metallic salts in some tattoo pigments may appear radiopaque
▶ Tangent (horizontal beam) mammography will confirm dermal location
  ▪ Correlation with physical exam helpful to confirm tattoo location

Management

▶ Annual screening mammography

Selected References/Further Reading

Bassett LW, et al. *Diagnosis of Diseases of the Breast*, 2nd ed. Philadelphia: WB Saunders Co., 2005:405.

Brown RC, et al. Tattoos simulating calcifications on xeroradiographs of the breast. *Radiology* 1981;138:583-584.

History

▶ 48-year-old woman with a mass detected on screening mammogram

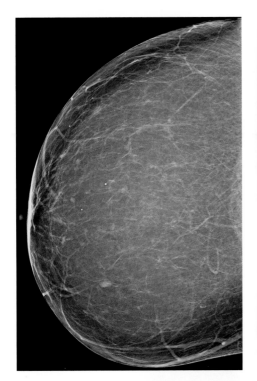 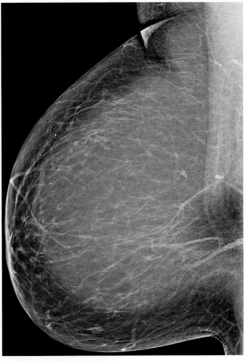

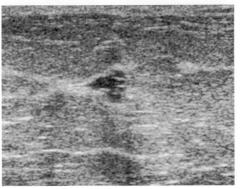

Case 61 Apocrine Metaplasia

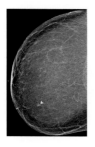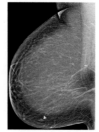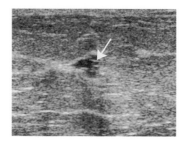

Findings

► Mammogram
  ▪ Lobular circumscribed low-density mass in the lower inner quadrant (*arrowheads*). No associated calcifications or distortion
► Ultrasound
  ▪ Clustered microcysts; note thin septa (*arrow*). No vascular flow was detected on Doppler imaging

Differential Diagnosis

► Fibrocystic change
► Complex cyst (when solid component suspected)

Teaching Points

► Common
  ▪ Women, ages 40s and 50s
► Small circumscribed lobular nodule with a corresponding cluster of simple cysts suggests apocrine metaplasia
  ▪ Ultrasound demonstrates tiny (2 to 3 mm) anechoic cysts with thin intervening septations
  ▪ No solid component
  ▪ High-frequency transducer required for optimal imaging
► Milk of calcium may coexist

Management

► Annual screening mammography
  ▪ When classic features present
► Short-term follow-up BI-RADS® Category 3
  ▪ When classic features are not optimally demonstrated on ultrasound
► Core needle biopsy is warranted when new, painful, enlarging, or solid component suspected
  ▪ Lower threshold in postmenopausal women
  ▪ Aspiration can be done; however, mass may not resolve due to the many septa

Selected References/Further Reading

Berg WA. Sonographically depicted breast clustered microcysts: is follow-up appropriate? *AJR* 2005;185:952-959.
Stavros AT. *Breast Ultrasound*. Philadelphia: Lippincott Williams & Wilkins, 2004; 93 and 186.
Warner JK, et al. Apocrine metaplasia: mammographic and sonographic appearances. *AJR* 1997;170:1375-1379.

History

▶ 32-year-old lactating woman with a new palpable mass

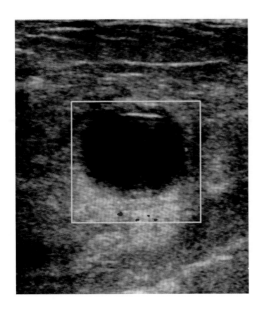

Case 62 Galactocele

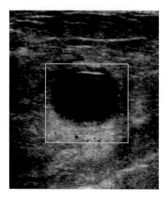

Findings

▸ Oval, nearly anechoic mass with posterior acoustic enhancement. No discernable internal vascular flow with Doppler imaging

Differential Diagnosis

▸ Simple cyst
▸ Complicated or complex cyst (if internal echoes present)

Teaching Points

▸ Focal collection of breast milk
▸ Uncommon
▸ Occurs in lactating females or patients who recently discontinued lactation
  ▪ Few reports described in female and male infants
▸ May mimic fibroadenoma or malignancy on clinical exam
▸ Mammogram appearance
  ▪ Typically a circumscribed, round or oval, equal-density mass
  ▪ Fat–fluid level may be seen on lateral view
    ◆ Most patients are imaged with ultrasound, so rarely seen in practice
  ▪ High lipid content may result in more radiolucent appearance
    ◆ Can mimic lipoma or hamartoma
▸ Ultrasound shows circumscribed, round or oval mass
  ▪ Anechoic or low-level internal echoes
    ◆ May have fluid–debris level
  ▪ May have internal echoes mimicking a solid component
    ◆ Consider aspiration to exclude a true complex mass

Management

▸ If uncertain of the diagnosis or if the patient is symptomatic, aspiration can be performed (but is not typically required)
  ▪ Demonstrates milk/milky fluid

Selected References/Further Reading

Bassett LW, et al. *Diagnosis of Diseases of the Breast*, 2nd ed. Philadelphia: WB Saunders Co., 2005:438-439.

Sabate JM, et al. Radiologic evaluation of breast disorders related to pregnancy and lactation. *RadioGraphics* 2007;27 Suppl 1:S101-24.

History

▶ Abnormal screening mammogram. Additional clinical history withheld. Left breast images shown

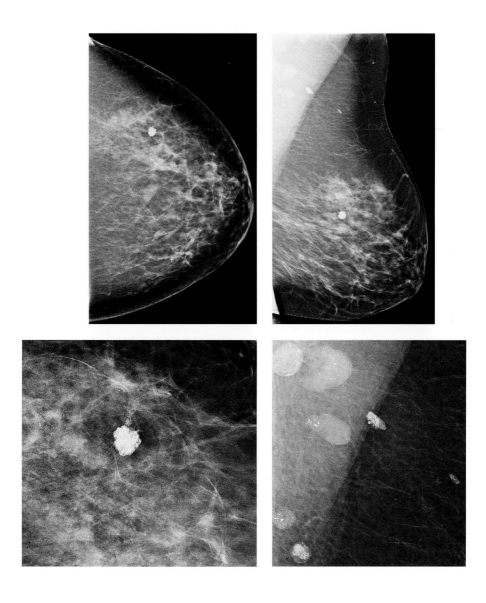

Case 63 Metastatic Ovarian Cancer to the Breast

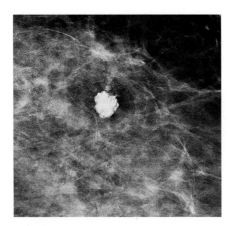 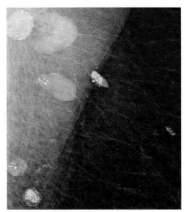

Findings

► Lobular, high-density mass with circumscribed margins and associated dense microcalcifications in the upper outer quadrant
  ▪ Magnified images show innumerable calcifications in multiple lymph nodes

Differential Diagnosis

► Metastatic breast carcinoma
► Silicone granuloma after implant rupture
► Granulomatous disease (e.g., tuberculosis, sarcoidosis)
► Metastatic thyroid carcinoma (rare)
► Gold particles from rheumatoid arthritis treatment (rare)

Teaching Points

► Metastasis of extra-mammary primary malignancy to the breast is uncommon
  ▪ Hematogenous spread
  ▪ Melanoma most common
    ♦ Dark tissue at core biopsy
► In this case, ovarian cancer (papillary serous adenocarcinoma) metastasized to an intramammary lymph node and axillary lymph nodes
  ▪ Poor prognosis
► Clinical history of known primary malignancy helpful

Management

► Ultrasound-guided core needle biopsy for diagnosis
► When diagnosis of metastatic disease confirmed, clinical management for primary malignancy
► Consider genetic counseling/testing
  ▪ BRCA gene mutations are associated with breast and ovarian cancer

Selected References/Further Reading

Bassett LW, et al. *Diagnosis of Diseases of the Breast*, 2nd ed. Philadelphia: WB Saunders Co., 2005:513-515.
Ikeda DM. *Breast Imaging: The Requisites*. Philadelphia: Elsevier Mosby, 2004:109.

History

▶ 55-year-old asymptomatic woman. Screening mammogram

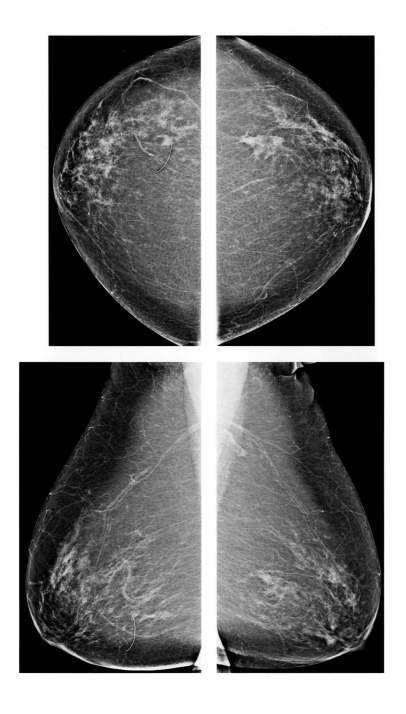

Case 64   Synchronous Bilateral Breast Cancer

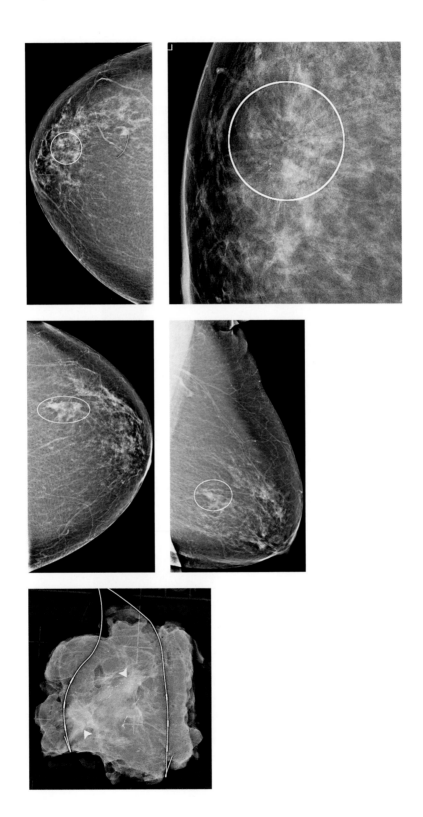

Findings

▶ Right breast: Subtle architectural distortion in the outer breast on the CC projection (*circle*), better demonstrated on the spot magnification CC view (*circle*)

▶ Left breast: Group of linear branching ("casting") microcalcifications in the upper outer quadrant (*circles*). The associated density is suspicious for an invasive component of malignancy (*arrowheads*) amidst ductal carcinoma in situ (best appreciated on specimen radiograph)

Differential Diagnosis

▶ Right breast
  ▪ Invasive lobular carcinoma (ILC)
  ▪ Invasive ductal carcinoma (IDC)
  ▪ Radial scar
▶ Left breast
  ▪ Invasive ductal carcinoma with extensive intraductal component
  ▪ Ductal carcinoma in situ (DCIS)

Teaching Points

▶ Synchronous bilateral breast cancer is uncommon
  ▪ Prevalence reported from 1% to 3%
▶ Has variable definitions in the literature
  ▪ Range includes as short as 3 months to as long as 12 months following the diagnosis of an index cancer
▶ Higher incidence with tumors having lobular histology (up to 30%)
▶ Higher risk for multifocal/multicentric disease
▶ Bilateral cancers may or may not have similar imaging features
▶ Genetic counseling should be considered in patients who present with bilateral cancer
  ▪ Higher risk for genetic disposition
▶ Resist satisfaction of search
  ▪ Lower your threshold for biopsy in patients with a known index cancer
    ◆ Both in the affected breast, and the contralateral breast

Management

▶ Bilateral image-guided percutaneous core needle biopsy for tissue diagnosis
▶ Consider contrast enhanced MR to evaluate extent of disease bilaterally

Selected References/Further Reading

Bassett LW, et al. *Diagnosis of Diseases of the Breast*, 2nd ed. Philadelphia: WB Saunders Co., 2005:509-510.
Lee SG, et al. MR imaging screening of the contralateral breast in patients with newly diagnosed breast cancer: Preliminary results. *Radiology* 2003;226:773-778.
Tabar L, et al. *Breast Cancer: The Art and Science of Early Detection with Mammography*. New York: Thieme, 2005:423-428.

History

▶ 58-year-old woman with a new palpable mass in the left breast. A metallic BB marks the area of concern

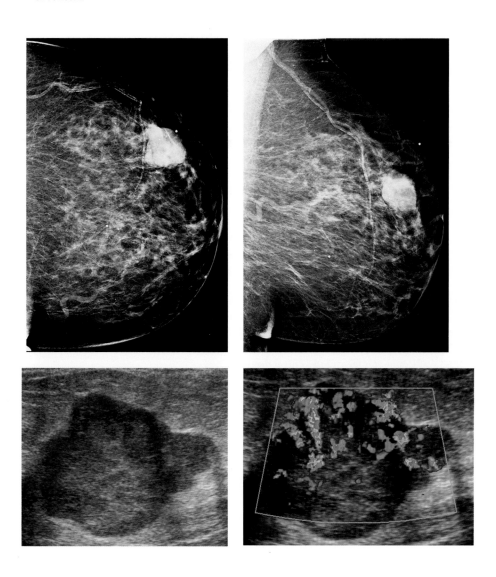

Case 65 Invasive Papillary Carcinoma

Findings

▶ Mammogram
  - High-density lobular mass with partially circumscribed, partially obscured margins. No associated calcifications. No associated architectural distortion
▶ Ultrasound
  - Lobular, hypoechoic, mass with circumscribed margins and marked increased vascularity on color Doppler imaging

Differential Diagnosis

▶ Invasive ductal carcinoma
▶ Phyllodes tumor
▶ Fibroadenoma (in younger patients)

Teaching Points

▶ Rare (approximately 0.5% of invasive breast cancers)
  - Mean age 65 years
  - Invasive carcinoma with exclusively papillary morphology
  - Pathologist must distinguish from other malignant papillary neoplasms
    ♦ Not the same entity as invasive *micro-papillary* carcinoma (IMPC)
      ∙ IMPC is more aggressive with poorer prognosis
▶ Classic presentation
  - Mammogram
    ♦ Solitary, predominantly circumscribed, high-density, round or oval mass, frequently in the central breast
    ♦ May have partially obscured or indistinct margin
    ♦ Commonly large (2 to 3 cm) at diagnosis
  - Ultrasound
    ♦ Solid or complex cystic mass with increased vascularity on color Doppler imaging
▶ Typically favorable prognosis

Management

▶ Ultrasound-guided core needle biopsy for tissue diagnosis
  - When presenting as a complex cystic mass, target the solid component for best sampling

Selected References/Further Reading

Berg W, et al. *Diagnostic Imaging Breast*. Salt Lake City, UT: Amirsys Inc., 2006: Part IV, Chapter 2, 170-173.

Collins LC, Schnitt SJ. Papillary lesions of the breast: Selected diagnostic and management issues. *Histopathology* 2008;53:20-29.

Pal SK, et al. Papillary carcinoma of the breast: an overview. *Breast Cancer Res Treat* 2010;122:637-645.

History

► Abnormal screening mammogram. Diagnostic mammogram and ultrasound images shown

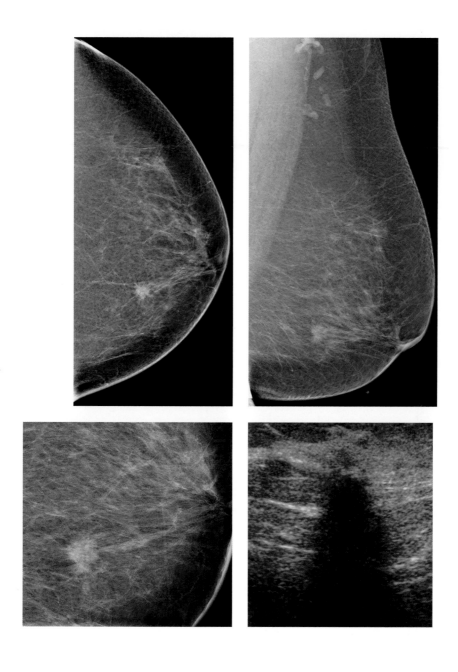

Case 66 Invasive Ductal Carcinoma with Extensive Intraductal Component (EIC)

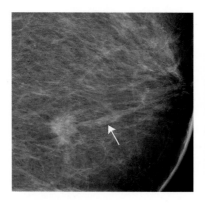 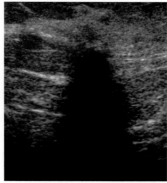

Findings

- ▶ Mammogram
  - ▪ High-density irregular mass with spiculated margins in lower inner left breast. A few faint calcifications are associated with the mass
  - ▪ Note the prominent duct anterior to the mass, suggesting intraductal extension (*arrow*)
- ▶ Ultrasound
  - ▪ Irregular hypoechoic mass with indistinct margins and marked posterior acoustic shadowing

Differential Diagnosis

- ▶ Ductal carcinoma in situ (less likely, given the presence of a mass)
- ▶ Invasive lobular carcinoma

Teaching Points

- ▶ Tumors are classified as having an *extensive intraductal component* (EIC) when
  - ▪ Predominantly intraductal, with small areas of invasion, or
  - ▪ Primarily invasive, with DCIS filling ducts within the invasive tumor, or
  - ▪ DCIS is present adjacent to the invasive tumor
- ▶ Associated with higher risk for local recurrence
- ▶ Evaluating extent of disease is important in surgical planning
  - ▪ Magnification views best depict extent of microcalcifications
- ▶ Classic mammographic appearance depicts a suspicious mass with associated and adjacent suspicious microcalcifications
  - ▪ Non-calcified DCIS can be mammographically occult
  - ▪ Tubular (ductal) density associated with a mass is suspicious (as in this case)
- ▶ Ultrasound may demonstrate findings of ductal extension
  - ▪ "Tail" of index mass extending into a duct
  - ▪ Hypoechoic material/mass within a dilated duct
- ▶ Resist satisfaction of search
  - ▪ Look carefully for associated calcifications and other masses when a suspicious abnormality is detected

Management

- ► Ultrasound-guided core biopsy for tissue diagnosis
  - ▪ When DCIS *and* invasive malignancy found on core biopsy, EIC probable
- ► Multiple wire localization ("bracket" needle localization) recommended to include the full extent of disease
- ► Close correlation with specimen radiograph required
- ► In cases with extensive microcalcifications, consider post-excision (pre-radiation) mammogram with magnification views of the surgical site, to document complete excision, even when surgical margins are histologically negative

Selected References/Further Reading

Bassett LW, et al. *Diagnosis of Diseases of the Breast*, 2nd ed. Philadelphia: WB Saunders Co., 2005:470-473.
Berg W, et al. *Diagnostic Imaging Breast*. Salt Lake City, UT: Amirsys Inc., 2006: Part V, Chapter 1, 14-17.
Stavros AT. *Breast Ultrasound*. Philadelphia: Lippincott Williams & Wilkins, 2004:635-638.
Tot T, et al. *Practical Breast Pathology*. New York: Thieme, 2002:147-149.

History

▶ Screening mammogram

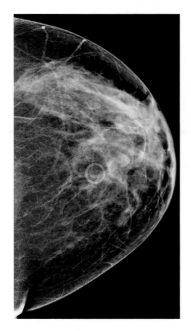 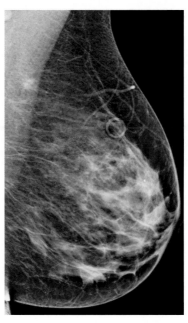

Case 67 Invasive Ductal Carcinoma as a One-view Finding

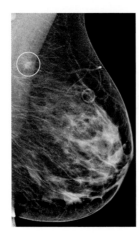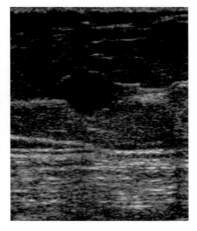

Findings

▶ Mammogram
  ▪ Focal asymmetry with architectural distortion in the upper breast, seen only on the MLO projection (larger white circle indicates the finding; the smaller circle is a mole marker placed on the skin)
  ▪ Could not be demonstrated on any CC projections
▶ Ultrasound
  ▪ Hypoechoic, irregular solid mass with angular margins in the upper inner quadrant (the entire upper breast was imaged in order to correlate with the one-view mammogram finding)

Differential Diagnosis

▶ Tubular carcinoma
▶ Radial scar (much less likely given ultrasound appearance)

Teaching Points

▶ Diagnostic evaluation was performed in an attempt to localize and characterize the initial finding (in this case exaggerated lateral CC and cleavage views were obtained)
  ▪ Tailored views may assist in localizing a one view finding in the orthogonal plane
  ▪ When a finding is seen on MLO but not CC, measure the posterior nipple line (PNL)
    ◆ PNL on CC view should be within 1 cm of PNL on MLO view. If not, then deep tissue excluded from CC view. Repeat CC or perform exaggerated views
▶ Asymmetry may be the only imaging feature of carcinoma on screening examinations
  ▪ One-view finding by definition
▶ Most asymmetries represent summation artifact

- Any new or developing asymmetry should be evaluated with diagnostic imaging
  - Especially in retroglandular fat, medial breast, subareolar breast
  - View with greater suspicion when associated with
    - Architectural distortion
    - Underlying solid mass
    - Microcalcifications
    - Or when *palpable*
- Comparing right and left breasts ("back-to-back") will help improve detection of masses that project over the pectoralis muscle
  - *Pitfall*: Mistaking a suspicious mass/asymmetry for a normal lymph node projecting over the pectoralis muscle on the MLO view

Management

- Ultrasound-guided core needle biopsy for tissue diagnosis

Selected References/Further Reading

Sickles EA. The spectrum of breast asymmetries: Imaging features, work-up, management. *Radiol Clin North Am* 2007;45:765-771.

Tabar L, et al. *Breast Cancer: The Art and Science of Early Detection with Mammography.* New York: Thieme, 2005:329-345.

History

▶ 63-year-old asymptomatic woman who underwent breast conservation therapy (BCT) four years ago. A spot magnification view of the lumpectomy site is shown

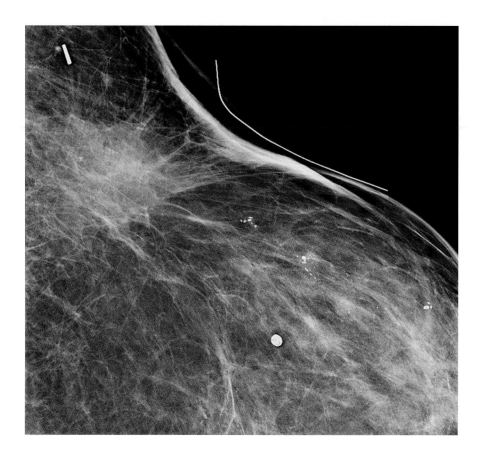

Case 68　Recurrent Ductal Carcinoma In Situ (DCIS)

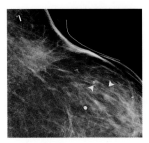

Findings

▶ Fine linear branching calcifications are noted anterior to the lumpectomy bed (*arrowheads*)

Differential Diagnosis

▶ Fat necrosis (highly unlikely in this case, given morphology of the calcifications)

Teaching Points

▶ Diagnostic mammography should be performed annually in patients who have undergone BCT
  ▪ In the first 5 years following BCT, magnification views of the lumpectomy bed should be performed
▶ More difficult to detect recurrent cancer in a treated breast due to
  ▪ Architectural distortion from surgery
  ▪ Radiation changes
▶ Fat necrosis commonly occurs in the lumpectomy bed
  ▪ Typically round, lucent center
  ▪ Typically develops more than 2 years post-treatment
  ▪ Careful analysis of the calcification morphology can allow discrimination between most benign and suspicious findings
    ◆ Biopsy indeterminate findings
▶ NSABP-B-60 (National Surgical Adjuvant Breast and Bowel Project) trial data
  ▪ 70% of ipsilateral recurrences occurred within 10 years of BCT
    ◆ 40% in the first 5 years
    ◆ 30% in the second 5 years
▶ Recurrence rarely occurs in the first 18 months following completion of therapy

Management

▶ Stereotactic core needle biopsy for tissue diagnosis
▶ Mastectomy recommended for patients with recurrent malignancy following BCT

Selected References/Further Reading

Bland K, Copeland E. *The Breast: Comprehensive Management of Benign and Malignant Disorders.* St. Louis, MOL Saunders, 2004: Chapter 43.

Fisher B, et al. Twenty-year follow-up of a randomized trial comparing total mastectomy, lumpectomy, and lumpectomy plus irradiation for the treatment of invasive breast cancer. *N Engl J Med* 2002;347:1233-1241.

Fisher B, et al. Treatment of lymph-node-negative, estrogen-receptor-positive breast cancer: long-term findings from National Surgical Adjuvant Breast and Bowel Project randomized clinical trials. *Lancet* 2004;364:820-821.

History

► New screen-detected mass in the left breast, lower inner quadrant. Spot magnification view and ultrasound are shown

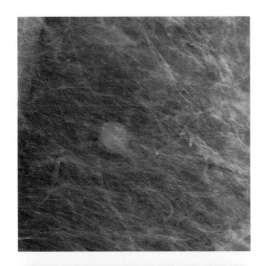

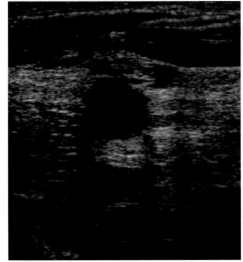

Case 69 Ductal Adenoma

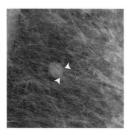 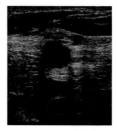

Findings

- ► Mammogram
  - ▪ Round, non-calcified, equal-density mass. Note the partially obscured border (*arrowheads*)
- ► Ultrasound
  - ▪ Round, hypoechoic, solid, circumscribed mass with mild posterior acoustic enhancement

Differential Diagnosis

- ► Fibroadenoma
- ► Lactating adenoma (in a pregnant or lactating female; typically presents as a palpable mass)
- ► Malignancy (high-grade invasive ductal carcinoma, mucinous carcinoma)

Teaching Points

- ► Also known as tubular adenoma
- ► Rare
- ► Benign
  - ▪ Related to fibroadenoma
- ► Typically encountered in younger patients
  - ▪ May present as a palpable mass on clinical exam
  - ▪ May be screen-detected in patients over 40 years
- ► Classic appearance
  - ▪ Mammogram
    - ◆ Round or oval, circumscribed mass
    - ◆ +/- calcifications
  - ▪ Ultrasound
    - ◆ Round or oval, circumscribed homogeneously hypoechoic mass
  - ▪ Similar imaging appearance to fibroadenoma in younger patients
  - ▪ May have indeterminate or suspicious features in older patients

Management

- ► BI-RADS® Category 4: Suspicious abnormality
- ► Ultrasound-guided core needle biopsy for tissue diagnosis

Selected References/Further Reading

Berg W, et al. *Diagnostic Imaging Breast*. Salt Lake City, UT: Amirsys Inc., 2006: Part IV, Chapter 2, 2-3.

Soo MS, et al. Tubular adenomas of the breast: Imaging findings with histologic correlation. *AJR* 2000;174:757-761.

History

▶ Baseline screening mammogram

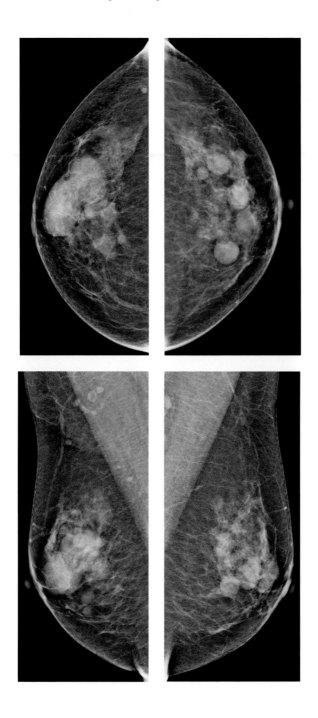

Case 70 Bilateral Benign-Appearing Masses (Rule of Multiplicity)

Findings

▶ Multiple, bilateral, round to oval, predominantly circumscribed, non-calcified equal-density masses

Differential Diagnosis

▶ Multiple bilateral benign cysts
▶ Multiple bilateral fibroadenomas

Teaching Points

▶ Multiple bilateral benign-appearing masses are most likely cysts or fibroadenomas
  ▪ No increased risk for breast cancer
▶ Diagnostic workup not required, as outlined below
▶ Criteria to invoke rule of multiplicity and assign BI-RADS® Category 2 assessment on screening examination
  ▪ At least three masses present (at least one mass in each breast)
  ▪ Circumscribed margins (more than 75% clearly visible)
    ♦ No indistinct or spiculated margins may be present
  ▪ No suspicious microcalcifications
  ▪ Masses must appear generally similar in shape, size, density
▶ Diagnostic evaluation REQUIRED when
  ▪ Any suspicious finding superimposed on bilateral benign-appearing masses
  ▪ Interval increase in size of one mass
    ♦ Or development of suspicious features
  ▪ *Palpable* mass present
▶ Multifocal/multicentric cancer is typically unilateral
  ▪ Critical that masses be *bilateral* in order to assign a benign assessment

Management

▶ BI-RADS® Category 2: Benign findings
▶ Annual screening mammography

Selected References/Further Reading

Berg W, et al. *Diagnostic Imaging Breast*. Salt Lake City, UT: Amirsys Inc., 2006: Part IV, Chapter 5, 22-25.
Leung JWT, Sickles EA. Multiple bilateral masses detected on screening mammography: assessment of need for recall imaging. *AJR* 2000;175:23-29.

History

▶ 54-year-old woman undergoing annual screening mammography. Additional clinical history withheld

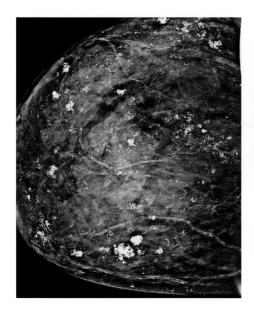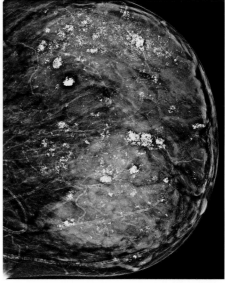

Case 71 Bilateral Benign Metastatic Calcifications in a Patient with Renal Failure and Hyperparathyroidism

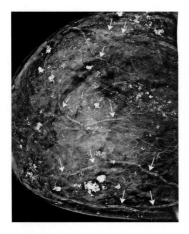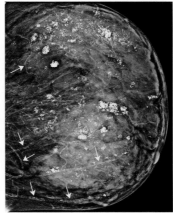

Findings

▶ Multiple, bilateral, coarse, diffuse calcifications superimposed on a background of punctuate and round diffuse calcifications

▶ Also note the extensive vascular calcifications (*arrows*)

Differential Diagnosis

▶ Dermatomyositis (produces extensive skin calcifications, which at first glance may have a similar appearance)

Teaching Points

▶ This case is an extremely extensive presentation of this diagnosis
▶ Chronic renal failure results in altered calcium metabolism
 ▪ Leads to secondary hyperparathyroidism
 ▪ Can result in metastatic soft tissue calcifications
 ◆ "Metastatic" in this context does not refer to a malignant or neoplastic process, but rather names the accumulation of calcium salts in previously healthy tissues
▶ Benign breast calcifications are very common in dialysis patients
 ▪ Vascular
 ▪ Stromal
 ▪ Secretory
 ▪ Skin
▶ Can occur in patients on dialysis or post-transplant

Management

▶ BI-RADS® Category 2: Benign findings
▶ Annual screening mammography

Selected References/Further Reading

Castellanos M, et al. Increased breast calcifications in women with end-stage renal disease on dialysis: implications for breast cancer screening. *Am J Kidney Dis* 2006;48:301-306.
Sommer G, et al. Breast calcifications in renal hyperparathyroidism. *AJR* 1987;148:855-857.

History

▶ 49-year-old woman with a history of atypical ductal hyperplasia (ADH) excised from the right breast upper outer quadrant three years ago. She was recalled from a screening mammogram for additional evaluation of new microcalcifications in the right breast. Spot magnification CC and ML views are shown

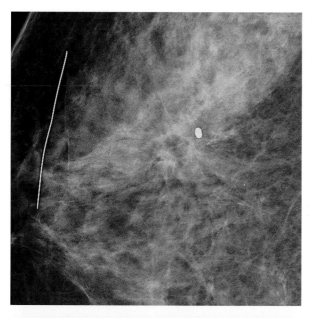

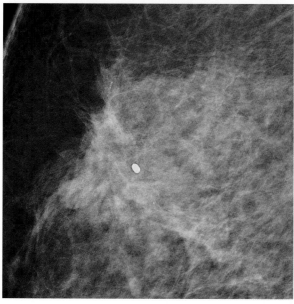

Case 72 Atypical Ductal Hyperplasia (ADH) at Site of Previous Excisional Biopsy for ADH

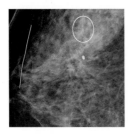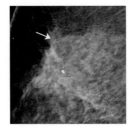

Findings

▸ Amorphous and indistinct microcalcifications on the CC view (*circle*)
▸ Calcifications appear to have a linear distribution on the lateral magnification view (*arrow*)
▸ Architectural distortion is attributed to previous excision and was stable mammographically

Differential Diagnosis

▸ Ductal carcinoma in situ (DCIS)
▸ Benign calcifications (adenosis, fibrocystic change)

Teaching Points

▸ ADH is a high-risk marker for breast cancer
  ▪ 4- to 5-fold increased relative risk
  ▪ Risk increased bilaterally
▸ ADH on core needle biopsy warrants surgical excisional biopsy
  ▪ Variable reports (10% to 25%) of upgrade to malignancy (DCIS or invasive carcinoma) at surgical excision
▸ ADH is most often found in association with amorphous calcifications
  ▪ May coexist with fibroadenomas or papillomas
▸ When ADH is present at surgical margins, re-excision is not required

Management

▸ Given this patient's history of ADH in the same quadrant previously, excisional biopsy was performed for diagnosis (in lieu of stereotactic core needle biopsy)
  ▪ Felt to be at high risk for additional ADH or DCIS
▸ Patient is at high risk for developing breast cancer
  ▪ Lower threshold for biopsy in high-risk patients
  ▪ Consider MR screening in conjunction with annual mammography
▸ Chemoprevention (e.g., Tamoxifen) may be considered for risk reduction

Selected References/Further Reading

Berg WA. Image-guided breast biopsy and management of high-risk lesions. *Radiol Clin North Am* 2004;42(5):935-946.
Berg WA, et al. Biopsy of amorphous breast calcifications: pathologic outcome and yield at stereotactic biopsy. *Radiology* 2001;221:495-503.
Greene T, et al. The significance of surgical margins for patients with atypical ductal hyperplasia. *Am J Surg* 2006;192:499-501.

History

▶ 55-year-old woman undergoing annual screening examination. Mammogram from 4 years ago shown for comparison (CC images shown)

Comparison from four years ago

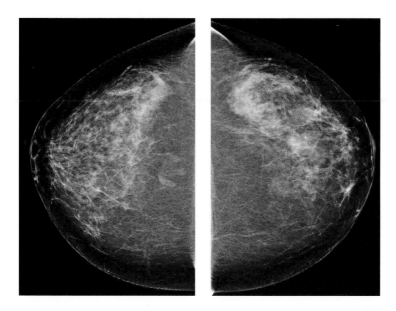

Current exam

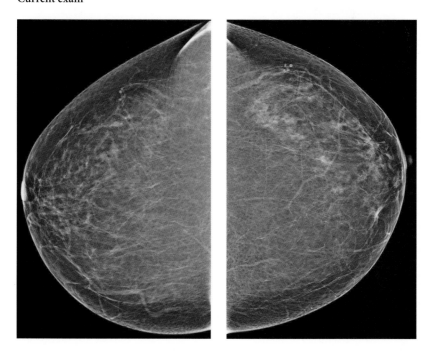

Case 73   Normal Fatty Involution of Breast Parenchyma

Findings

▶ Bilateral, symmetric, decrease in overall glandular tissue (fatty replacement) since the previous examination. No suspicious finding in either breast

Differential Diagnosis

▶ Significant weight gain (increase in fatty tissue)

▶ Incorrect patient (consider this when there is a dramatic difference in the overall appearance of exams)

▶ Reduction mammoplasty (may result in decreased density, but associated postoperative findings would be present)

Teaching Points

▶ All mammogram reports should contain a description of breast parenchymal density
  ▪ Four described densities (BI-RADS® terminology)
    ◆ Almost entirely fat (<25% glandular)
    ◆ Scattered fibroglandular densities (25% to 50% glandular)
    ◆ Heterogeneously dense (51% to 75% glandular)
    ◆ Extremely dense (>75% glandular)

▶ Mammographic density is affected by multiple factors
  ▪ Age
  ▪ Hormonal status
  ▪ Genetics
  ▪ Weight fluctuations

▶ Sensitivity of mammography is inversely related to density: as density increases, sensitivity decreases

▶ Generally, parenchymal density is inverse to age
  ▪ Younger women have denser breasts
  ▪ Fatty replacement occurs with advancing age

▶ Increasing parenchymal density is commonly observed when patients are
  ▪ Pregnant/lactating
  ▪ Taking exogenous hormone replacement therapy (HRT)

Management

▶ Annual screening mammography

Selected References/Further Reading

American College of Radiology (ACR). ACR BI-RADS®—Mammography, 4th ed. *ACR Breast Imaging Reporting and Data Systems, Breast Imaging Atlas.* Reston, VA: American College of Radiology, 2003:179-189.

Bassett LW, et al. *Diagnosis of Diseases of the Breast*, 2nd ed. Philadelphia: WB Saunders Co., 2005: Chapter 24.

Berg W, et al. *Diagnostic Imaging Breast.* Salt Lake City, UT: Amirsys Inc., 2006: Part IV, Chapter 5, 48-49.

History

► Food and Drug Administration (FDA) inspection next week

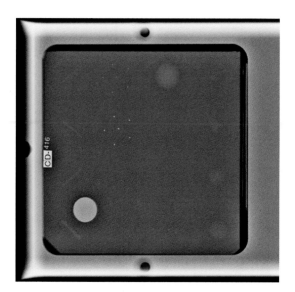

Case 74   Phantom Imaging for Quality Assurance

Findings

▶ Digital image of American College of Radiology (ACR) phantom within acceptable parameters

Differential Diagnosis

▶ Variable depending on appearance of phantom

Teaching Points

▶ Mammography Quality Standards Act (MQSA) of 1992 requires mammography facilities to be accredited, certified, and inspected
  ▪ Illegal to practice mammography without a current MQSA certificate
  ▪ Facility is subject to annual FDA inspection
    ◆ Or state certifying body
▶ ACR is an MQSA-approved accreditation body
  ▪ Phantom imaging for ACR accreditation performed with dosimeter
    ◆ Reviewed by ACR physicists
▶ Phantom imaging is required weekly
  ▪ Images kept for annual inspection
  ▪ Tests performance of the imaging system
    ◆ Quantitative evaluation of unit's ability to image small structures similar to those found *in vivo*
  ▪ Materials embedded within the phantom simulate
    ◆ Calcifications
    ◆ Tumor masses
▶ Digital and analog mammography systems must score the following on phantom images
  ▪ Four fibers
  ▪ Three speck groups
  ▪ Three masses
▶ FDA requires facilities with digital mammography to follow the quality control (QC) manual from the manufacturer
  ▪ Each manufacturer has specific QC program for test frequencies and parameters
▶ Every facility must have a lead interpreting physician to oversee quality assurance (QA) program
  ▪ Consult lead QC technologist and medical physicist when questions or problems arise

Management

▶ Perform QC in accordance with FDA/MQSA guidelines
▶ FDA website for up-to-date information is http://www.fda.gov/Radiation-EmittingProducts/MammographyQualityStandardsActandProgram/default.htm

Selected References/Further Reading

American College of Radiology. *Mammography Quality Control Manual*. Reston, VA: American College of Radiology, 1999.

Bassett LW, et al. *Diagnosis of Diseases of the Breast*, 2nd ed. Philadelphia: WB Saunders Co., 2005: Chapter 6.

Mammography Quality Standards Act of 1992, Public Law No. 102-539.

History

► Screening mammogram

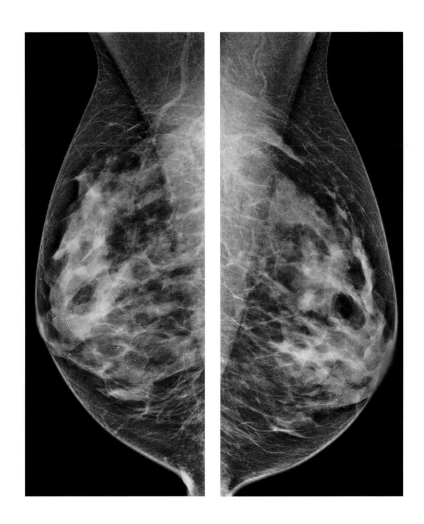

Case 75   Bilateral Benign Calcifications

Findings

▶ Innumerable, bilateral, diffusely scattered, punctate and round microcalcifications

Differential Diagnosis

▶ Imaging artifact (analog mammography)
▶ Mimics of calcifications
  ▪ Talc
  ▪ Antiperspirant

Teaching Points

▶ Bilateral diffuse benign calcifications are commonly attributed to
  ▪ Adenosis
  ▪ Sclerosing adenosis
  ▪ Fibrocystic change
▶ Analysis of morphology and distribution critical to appropriate management of calcifications
  ▪ Diffuse, bilateral benign-appearing calcifications do not require diagnostic workup or biopsy
  ▪ If new, focal, grouped, or clustered, then additional evaluation with magnification mammography is recommended
▶ Patients with benign calcifications can develop malignancy
  ▪ Look carefully for morphologically suspicious calcifications superimposed on a background of benign calcifications
  ▪ Extensive calcifications may raise suspicion for ductal carcinoma in situ (DCIS) when
    ◆ Unilateral and morphologically suspicious
    ◆ Segmental rather than diffuse distribution
  ▪ Most suspicious feature directs management

Management

▶ BI-RADS® Category 2: Benign findings
▶ Annual screening mammography

Selected References/Further Reading

American College of Radiology (ACR). ACR BI-RADS®—Mammography, 4th ed. *ACR Breast Imaging Reporting and Data Systems, Breast Imaging Atlas*. Reston, VA: American College of Radiology, 2003:74-75.

Bassett LW, et al. *Diagnosis of Diseases of the Breast*, 2nd ed. Philadelphia: WB Saunders Co., 2005:439-442.

Sickles EA. Breast calcifications: mammographic evaluation. *Radiology* 1986;160:289-293.

History

▶ Abnormal screening mammogram. Spot magnification views of new microcalcifications in the left breast are shown

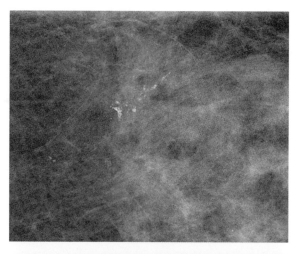

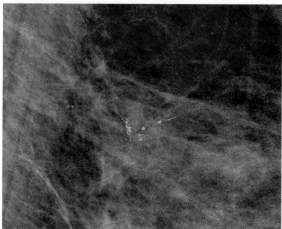

Case 76   Ductal Carcinoma In Situ (Intermediate-Grade)

Findings

▶ Clustered pleomorphic microcalcifications with associated linear ("casting") calcifications

Differential Diagnosis

▶ Invasive ductal carcinoma

Teaching Points

▶ DCIS is graded as low, intermediate, high
  ▪ Intermediate grade refers to low nuclear grade with focal necrosis
▶ Classically presents as calcifications on screening mammogram
  ◆ Pleomorphic
  ◆ Amorphous/indistinct
  ◆ Fine linear branching
  ▪ Occasionally has associated mass/density
    ◆ Consider ultrasound when density present
    ◆ May represent an invasive component of malignancy
    ◆ Ultrasound-guided core needle biopsy may be feasible
▶ Careful diagnostic evaluation required to evaluate extent of disease
  ▪ Magnification views may reveal additional suspicious calcifications
  ▪ Assists in surgical planning
▶ Difficult to distinguish grade by imaging, and is clinically unnecessary
  ▪ Pathologic determination made at time of core biopsy/excision
▶ When extensive calcifications are present, multiple wire localization ("bracket" needle localization) is recommended to include the full extent of disease
  ▪ Close correlation with specimen radiograph required
  ▪ Consider post-excision (pre-radiation) mammogram with magnification views of the surgical site, to document complete excision, even when surgical margins are histologically negative

Management

▶ Stereotactic core needle biopsy for tissue diagnosis
  ▪ Given the highly suspicious imaging features in this case, any core needle biopsy result yielding benign histology would be considered *discordant*
    ◆ Discordant biopsy results require surgical excision

Selected References/Further Reading

Bassett LW, et al. *Diagnosis of Diseases of the Breast*, 2nd ed. Philadelphia: WB Saunders Co., 2005: Chapter 26.
Sickles EA. Breast calcifications: mammographic evaluation. *Radiology* 1986;160:289-293.
Silverstein MJ, et al. Ductal carcinoma in situ: USC/Van Nuys Prognostic Index and the impact of margin status. *Breast* 2003;12:457-471.

History

▶ 52-year-old woman with a new palpable mass in the left breast. A metallic BB marks the area of concern

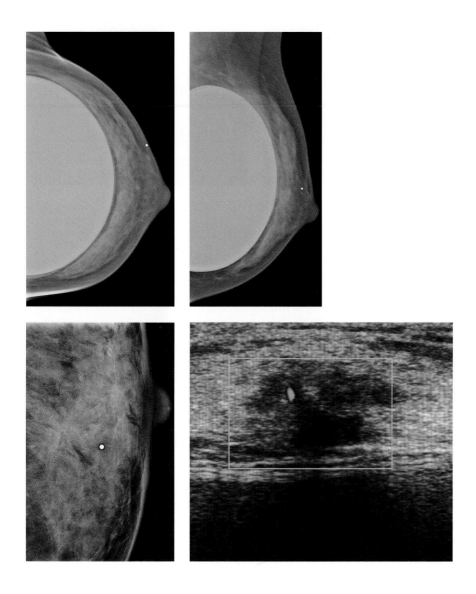

Case 77 Invasive Ductal Carcinoma (Grade 2) and Ductal Carcinoma In Situ (Low-Grade) in a Patient with Implants

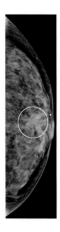 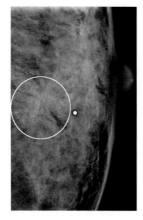 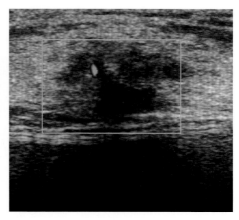

Findings

▶ Mammogram
  ▪ A subpectoral silicone implant present
  ▪ No discernable abnormality is present on the standard views
  ▪ The MLO implant-displaced and spot ML magnification views demonstrate architectural distortion corresponding with the palpable mass (*circles*)
▶ Ultrasound
  ▪ Irregular, hypoechoic mass with indistinct margins and increased vascular flow

Differential Diagnosis

▶ Invasive lobular carcinoma

Teaching Points

▶ Implants can make performing and interpreting mammography more challenging
  ▪ Limit visualization of parenchyma
  ▪ Make it difficult to achieve adequate compression
    ◆ Compression may be painful when capsular contracture present
▶ When mammography is performed correctly, risk of implant damage is extremely low
▶ Standard CC, MLO, and "implant-displaced" CC and MLO (also known as Eklund or "push-back") views must be performed
  ▪ Note in this case how the mass is imperceptible on the standard (non-implant displaced) views
▶ In symptomatic patients with implants, increase reliance on and utilization of ultrasound (US) in conjunction with mammography
  ▪ Even when fatty replaced on mammogram

- Directed US will ensure that a palpable mass is not obscured by the implant mammographically
- Palpable mass(es) may represent silicone from extracapsular implant rupture

Management

▶ Ultrasound-guided core needle biopsy for tissue diagnosis
  ▪ Obtain informed consent for possible implant rupture
  ▪ Careful attention to positioning and needle placement is necessary during the biopsy to avoid damaging the underlying implant
  ▪ Consider using a cutting needle without a "throw" for increased control
  ▪ Inject local anesthetic posterior to the mass to increase distance between the target and underlying implant
  ▪ Rarely, percutaneous core needle biopsy may not be technically feasible in patients with implants
    - Consider fine-needle aspiration or surgical excision for diagnosis when appropriate

Selected References/Further Reading

Fornage BD, Sneige N, Singletary SE. Masses in breasts with implants: diagnosis with US-guided fine-needle aspiration biopsy. *Radiology* 1994;191:339-342.

Middleton MS, McNamara MP. *Breast Implant Imaging*. Philadelphia: Lippincott Williams & Wilkins, 2003: Chapter 11.

Parker SH, Klaus AJ. Performing a breast biopsy with a directional, vacuum-assisted biopsy instrument. *RadioGraphics* 1997;17:1233-1252.

History

▶ A 33-year-old woman with a new palpable mass in the right medial breast

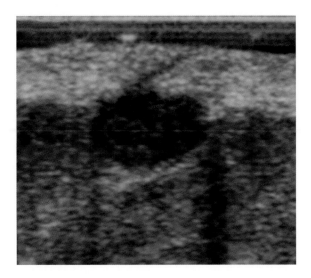

Case 78   Sebaceous Cyst

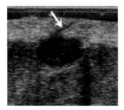

Findings

- ▶ Superficial, homogeneously hypoechoic, oval mass without internal vascular flow
- ▶ Note the tract extending from the mass to the skin surface (*arrow*)

Differential Diagnosis

- ▶ Epidermal inclusion cyst (caused by surgery, biopsy, or penetrating trauma)
- ▶ Superficial abscess
- ▶ Montgomery gland cyst (if periareloar location)

Teaching Points

- ▶ Superficial, often palpable, cutaneous or subcutaneous epithelial cyst
  - ▪ Contains sebaceous glands
- ▶ Clinically presents as
  - ▪ A palpable mass
  - ▪ Often with a visible punctum or "blackhead" at the skin surface
  - ▪ May be erythematous and tender when inflamed/infected
  - ▪ More commonly seen in cleavage/medial breast and axilla
- ▶ May be entirely in the skin, partially subcutaneous, or mostly subcutaneous with a small tract connecting out to the skin surface
  - ▪ Partially subcutaneous may demonstrate "claw sign"
    - ◆ Hyperechoic skin seen around the subcutaneous portion of the lesion
  - ▪ Deep lesions may show gland neck/tract to skin (as in this case)
- ▶ Imaging evaluation
  - ▪ Tangential magnification views may show relationship to skin to best advantage
  - ▪ Ultrasound helpful to demonstrate classic findings (as seen in this case)
    - ◆ Imaging with standoff pad or extra gel helpful to see tract
    - ◆ Increased peripheral vascularity common when inflamed
- ▶ Important to differentiate from a breast parenchymal neoplasm
  - ▪ Caveat: Do not mistake a superficial suspicious mass for a sebaceous cyst

Management

- ▶ Very conservative except when infected
  - ▪ BI-RADS® Category 2 assessment when classic features are present
- ▶ Aspiration is not helpful
  - ▪ Thick material may not aspirate, or may reaccumulate
  - ▪ May precipitate infection or inflammation
- ▶ Can be surgically excised if clinically indicated

Selected References/Further Reading

Berg W, et al. *Diagnostic Imaging Breast.* Salt Lake City, UT: Amirsys Inc., 2006: Part IV, Chapter 3, 16-22.

Stavros AT. *Breast Ultrasound.* Philadelphia: Lippincott Williams & Wilkins, 2004:325-333.

History

▶ 62 year-old woman with a palpable mass in the left breast. A metallic BB denotes the area of concern

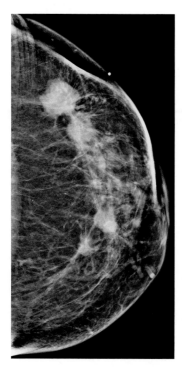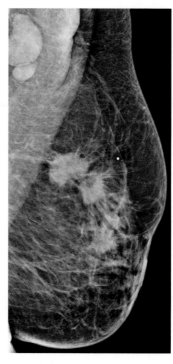

Case 79 Multicentric Invasive Ductal Carcinoma

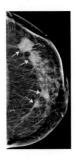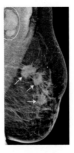

Findings

▶ Irregular high-density mass with spiculated margins in the upper outer quadrant corresponding to the palpable mass
▶ Multiple additional similar-appearing masses (*arrows*) extend into the upper inner quadrant
▶ Note the extensive lymphadenopathy (*circle*)

Differential Diagnosis

▶ None—classic appearance demonstrated

Teaching Points

▶ Multicentric (MC) disease involves more than two foci of malignancy in different quadrants (or >5 cm total involvement)
  ▪ True MC disease is uncommon
▶ Multifocal (MF) disease involves more than two foci of malignancy in the same quadrant
▶ Significant treatment and prognostic implications
  ▪ MC disease typically precludes breast conservation therapy
  ▪ Patients with either MF and/or MC disease are at increased risk for local recurrence
▶ Lower threshold for additional biopsies of findings in the affected breast
  ▪ "Incidental" lesions with "probably benign" findings more likely to be malignant
▶ Resist satisfaction of search

Management

▶ Ultrasound-guided core needle biopsy of two distinct masses for tissue diagnosis and to document full extent of disease
▶ Ultrasound-guided fine-needle aspiration (FNA) of the most suspicious axillary lymph node
  ▪ If the lymph node FNA yields metastatic disease, then sentinel lymph node sampling is not performed; the patient would undergo axillary lymph node dissection
▶ Consider MR for additional screening of the contralateral breast
▶ Mastectomy was performed

Selected References/Further Reading

Bassett LW, et al. *Diagnosis of Diseases of the Breast*, 2nd ed. Philadelphia: WB Saunders Co., 2005: Chapter 27.
Berg WA, Gilbreath PL. Multicentric and multifocal cancer: whole-breast ultrasound in preoperative evaluation. *Radiology* 2000;21:59-66.
Bland K, Copeland E. *The Breast: Comprehensive Management of Benign and Malignant Disorders*. St. Louis, MO: Saunders, 2004: Chapter 13.

History

▶ Abnormal screening mammogram. Select diagnostic mammographic images of the right breast shown

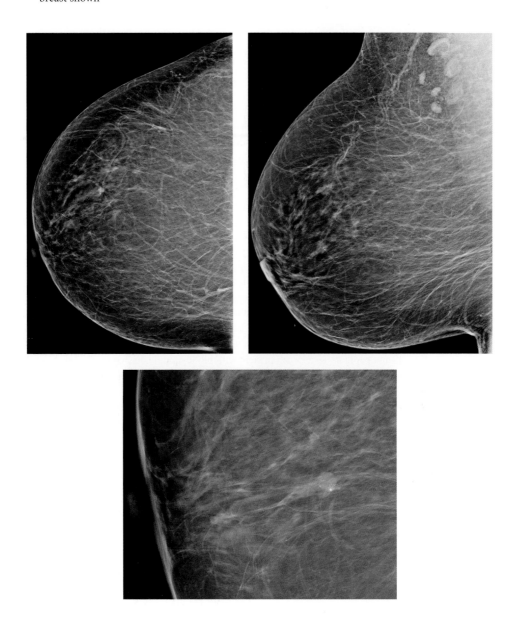

Case 80   Ductal Carcinoma In Situ (DCIS) Arising in a Papilloma

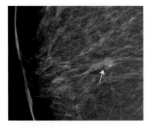

Findings

▶ Round, partially circumscribed, partially obscured (*arrow*), equal-density mass with associated heterogeneous microcalcifications

Differential Diagnosis

▶ Benign papilloma
▶ Atypical papilloma
▶ Invasive ductal carcinoma

Teaching Points

▶ Papillary lesions of any type (benign, atypical, or malignant) are relatively rare
  ▪ May represent as many as 5% of biopsied lesions, but many series report fewer
▶ Papillary lesions occur within the lactiferous ducts
  ▪ Composed of frond-like excrescences of tissue consisting of a fibrovascular core or stalk lined with an inner myoepithelial cell layer and an outer epithelial cell layer
▶ Papillary lesions confer an increased risk of breast cancer
▶ Both DCIS and papillary lesions can present with bloody nipple discharge
▶ Difficult to distinguish benign or malignant papillary features pathologically

Management

▶ Ultrasound-guided or stereotactic core needle biopsy for tissue diagnosis
  ▪ If a papillary lesion is suspected prospectively, extensive tissue sampling recommended
  ▪ Universal agreement to excise papillary lesions with associated atypia or malignancy found at core needle biopsy (CNB)
  ▪ However, a CNB resulting in a "benign" papilloma may result in atypia or malignancy upon excisional
    ◆ Reports vary as to how many patients are "upgraded" on excision biopsy to atypia or malignancy (range from 0% to 25%)
    ◆ Careful correlation between imaging and biopsy results recommended
      • If the radiologist or pathologist are uncertain, or discordant result, recommend excision

Selected References/Further Reading

Collins LC, Schnitt SJ. Papillary lesions of the breast: selected diagnostic and management issues. *Histopathology* 2008;52:20-29.

Mulligan AM, O'Malley FP. Papillary lesions of the breast: a review. *Adv Anat Pathol* 2007;14(2):108-119.

Rizzo M, et al. Surgical follow-up and clinical presentation of 142 breast papillary lesions diagnosed by ultrasound-guided core-needle biopsy. *Ann Surg Oncol* 2008;15:1040-1047.

History

▶ Screening mammogram

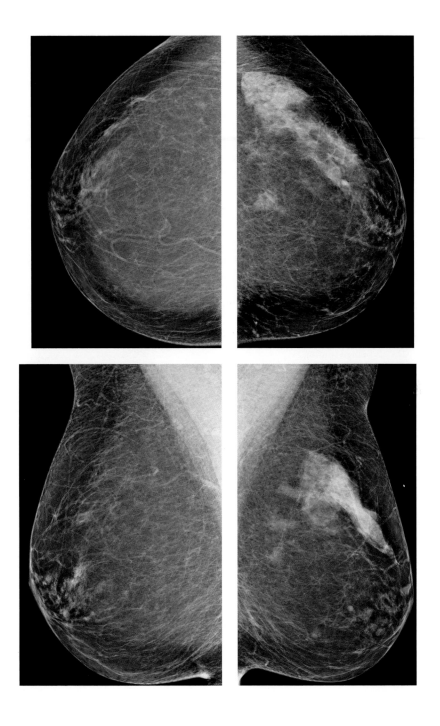

Case 81   Global Asymmetric Breast Tissue—Normal Variant

Findings

▶ Asymmetric glandular tissue involving the entire left upper outer quadrant. No mass, architectural distortion, or calcifications present

Differential Diagnosis

▶ Pseudoangiomatous stromal hyperplasia (PASH)
▶ Invasive lobular carcinoma (when global asymmetry is new or developing)

Teaching Points

▶ Global asymmetry by definition involves a quadrant, or more, of the breast
  ▪ Previously known as "asymmetric breast tissue"
▶ Asymmetric fibroglandular tissue more pronounced in one breast than the other
  ▪ Typically a normal variant
  ▪ Concave outward borders
    ◆ Distinguishes from a mass
  ▪ Interspersed with fat
  ▪ Frequently involves the upper outer quadrant
  ▪ No mass or architectural distortion present
  ▪ Visible on both views (unlike focal asymmetry)
▶ Less concerning than a focal asymmetry
▶ If corresponds with palpable mass, diagnostic mammography and ultrasound required

Management

▶ BI-RADS® 2: Benign finding
  ▪ When encountered at screening (non-palpable finding), very low probability of malignancy
    ◆ Such a dramatic finding would be palpable if malignant
  ▪ Therefore, annual screening mammography recommended
▶ Comparison with previous films always helpful
  ▪ If new or developing, biopsy should be considered

Selected References/Further Reading

American College of Radiology (ACR). ACR BI-RADS®—Mammography, 4th ed. *ACR Breast Imaging Reporting and Data Systems, Breast Imaging Atlas*. Reston, VA: American College of Radiology, 2003:146-149, 253-254.

Sickles EA. The spectrum of breast asymmetries: imaging features, work-up, management. *Radiol Clin North Am* 2007;45:765-771.

History

► 54-year-old woman undergoing screening mammogram (Select 90° lateral magnification mammography images included)

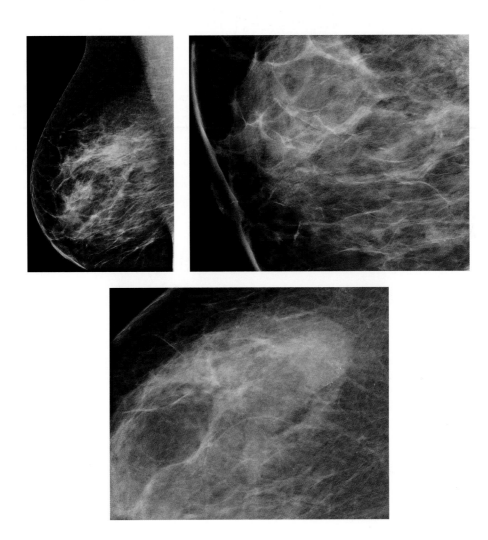

Case 82 Multicentric Ductal Carcinoma In Situ (DCIS)

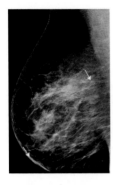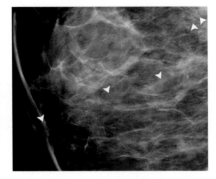

Findings

- ▶ Extensive calcifications are present in the right breast
  - ▪ Grouped pleomorphic calcifications are present in the deep breast (*arrow*)
  - ▪ Faint linear calcifications extend anteriorly to the nipple (*arrowheads*) spanning a total distance of 7 cm

Differential Diagnosis

- ▶ DCIS with invasive ductal carcinoma (IDC)

Teaching Points

- ▶ Multicentric disease involves
  - ▪ more than two foci of malignancy in different quadrants or
  - ▪ more than 5 cm total involvement
- ▶ When biopsy-proven extent of disease exceeds 5 cm most patients are not considered candidates for breast conserving surgery
  - ▪ Multiple biopsies may be required to prove extent of disease
- ▶ When extensive suspicious microcalcifications are present, ultrasound can be performed to possibly identify an underlying or obscured mass (especially in patients with dense breast parenchyma)
  - ▪ Proving the presence of invasive disease helps direct surgical management
    - ◆ If present on core biopsy, patients undergo sentinel lymph node biopsy at the time of lumpectomy

Management

- ▶ Stereotactic core needle biopsy for tissue diagnosis
  - ▪ Multiple sites biopsied to prove extent
  - ▪ Choose most suspicious sites, which are furthest apart, to assist in surgical planning
- ▶ Mastectomy for definitive treatment

Selected References/Further Reading

Bassett LW, et al. *Diagnosis of Diseases of the Breast*, 2nd ed. Philadelphia: WB Saunders Co., 2005: Chapter 26.

Sickles EA. Breast calcifications: mammographic evaluation. *Radiology* 1986;160:289-293.

Silverstein MJ. *Ductal Carcinoma In Situ of the Breast*, 2nd ed. Philadelphia: Lippincott Williams & Wilkins, 2002: Chapter 10.

History

► New palpable mass in the right breast. The patient reports recent trauma to the right breast with subsequent bruising. A metallic BB denotes the area of concern

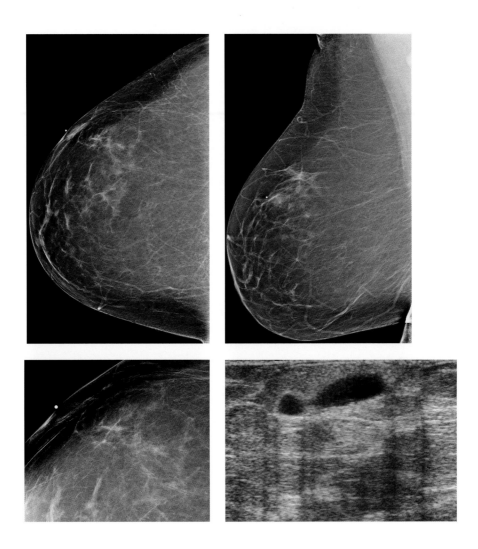

Case 83 Hematoma

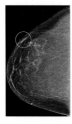 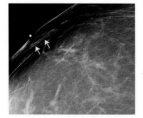

Findings

- ▶ Mammogram
  - ▪ Vague focal asymmetry in upper outer right breast (*circle*) in the area of palpable concern
  - ▪ Tangential view confirms superficial location of the lesion (*arrows*)
- ▶ Ultrasound
  - ▪ Fluid-containing, heterogeneous, oval superficial mass with echogenic wall

Differential Diagnosis

- ▶ Oil cysts/fat necrosis
- ▶ Cysts
- ▶ Intra-cystic neoplasm with hemorrhage

Teaching Points

- ▶ Collection of blood in breast tissue
- ▶ History is important in making correct diagnosis
- ▶ May be due to any blunt force or penetrating trauma
  - ▪ The patient may not recall a specific traumatic event
- ▶ Mammography may demonstrate a mass or new density with mixed tissue and fat
- ▶ Ultrasound appearance will depend on stage
  - ▪ Anechoic (fluid), solid (clot), or heterogeneous (both)
  - ▪ May have thick echogenic wall
  - ▪ Posterior acoustic enhancement common
  - ▪ Occasionally fluid–debris level
- ▶ Fat necrosis may develop with time
  - ▪ Oil cysts
  - ▪ Calcifications

Management

- ▶ Clinical exam and history helpful to avoid misdiagnosis
- ▶ Conservative management and follow-up to complete clinical and/or imaging resolution
  - ▪ Rarely, a neoplasm may present with hemorrhage that obscures an underlying mass
    - ◆ When a mass persists on clinical exam, short-term imaging follow-up will ensure that an underlying suspicious mass was not obscured
  - ▪ If symptoms/mass resolve clinically, follow-up imaging is not required

Selected References/Further Reading

Bassett LW, et al. *Diagnosis of Diseases of the Breast*, 2nd ed. Philadelphia: WB Saunders Co., 2005:409-419.
Stavros AT. *Breast Ultrasound*. Philadelphia: Lippincott Williams & Wilkins, 2004:406-409.

History

▶ 34-year-old woman who reports spontaneous right bloody nipple discharge. She underwent prior benign excisional biopsy 2 years ago (results of biopsy withheld)

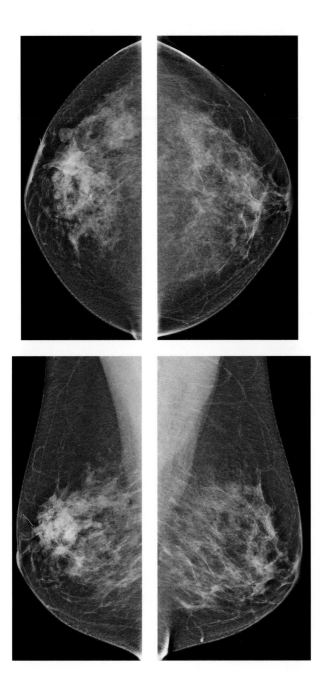

Case 84 Multiple Papillomas/Papillomatosis

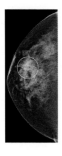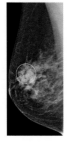

Findings

► Global asymmetry in the right breast
► Multiple round and tubular densities are present throughout the right breast
► A scar marker corresponds with architectural distortion (*circles*) from the prior benign excisional biopsy (which demonstrated papillomatosis)

Differential Diagnosis

► Multifocal invasive ductal carcinoma with intraductal extension
► Extensive duct ectasia (unlikely)
► Asymmetric cysts (unlikely)

Teaching Points

► "Papillomatosis" indicates multiple papillomas
  ▪ Can also refer to a pathologic diagnosis of microscopic foci of intraductal hyperplasia without atypia
► Commonly presents with pathologic nipple discharge
  ▪ Spontaneous or serous bloody nipple discharge from a single duct orifice
  ▪ Galactography/ductography can be helpful for imaging evaluation
  ▪ Ductoscopy (performed by some surgeons) is frequently diagnostic
► Papillary lesions of any type (benign, atypical, or malignant) are relatively rare
  ▪ May represent up to 5% of biopsied lesions, but many series report fewer
► Papillary lesions are associated with an increased risk of breast cancer
  ▪ Having multiple papillomas confers a greater risk than a single papilloma

Management

► Ultrasound-guided or stereotactic core needle biopsy for tissue diagnosis at the time of initial presentation
  ▪ This patient has known papillomatosis and is followed closely with clinical and imaging surveillance
  ▪ If there is interval change on imaging, repeat biopsy may be warranted
► After appropriate treatment (which may include surgical excision), careful screening follow-up is warranted, given the increased risk for breast cancer

Selected References/Further Reading

Ibarra JA. Papillary lesions of the breast. *Breast J* 2006;12(3):237-251.
Jung S-Y, et al. Risk factors for malignancy in benign papillomas of the breast on core needle biopsy. *World J Surg* 2010;34:261-265.
Lewis JT, et al. An analysis of breast cancer risk in women with single, multiple and atypical papilloma. *Am J Surg Pathol* 2006;30:665-672.

History

▶ Screening mammogram. Bilateral MLO views shown

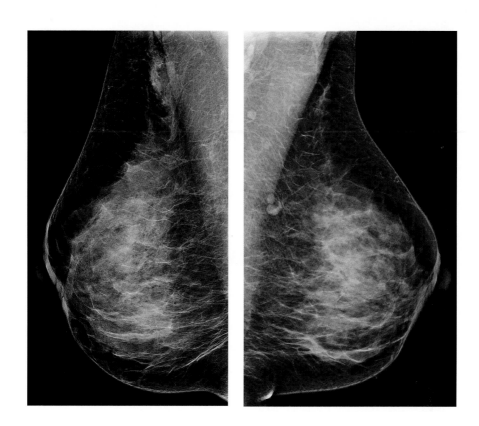

Case 85 Axillary Breast Tissue—Normal Variant

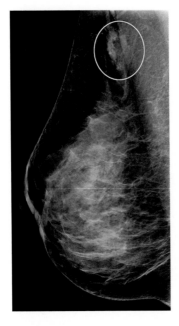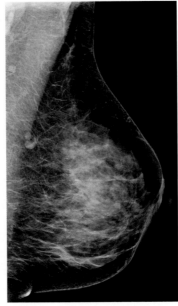

Findings

▸ Density that resembles normal-appearing glandular breast tissue projecting over the axilla on the MLO view (*circle*)
  ▪ Note there is no architectural distortion, mass, or suspicious microcalcifications

Differential Diagnosis

▸ None—classic appearance demonstrated
▸ *Caveat*: Do not dismiss a new or developing density or suspicious mass as normal axillary breast tissue

Teaching Points

▸ Aberrant or accessory breast tissue separate from the glandular tissue in the breast
  ▪ Results from incomplete involution of the mammary streak during embryonic development
  ▪ Distinct from the "tail of Spence," which is contiguous with the upper outer quadrant tissue
  ▪ Usually seen on the MLO view
  ▪ May be unilateral or bilateral
    ◆ Right > left reported
▸ Typically asymptomatic
  ▪ May present during pregnancy or with engorgement postpartum
  ▪ May present with cyclical pain
  ▪ May result in cosmetic concern for the patient

- ▶ Subject to same pathology as normally located breast tissue
  - ▪ Rare reports of fibroadenoma or cancer
    - ◆ Breast cancer can develop in any breast tissue
- ▶ A spectrum of aberrant clinical findings can exist along the "milk line" or mammary line (a line extending from the axillary region to the groin along which breast tissue can form)
  - ▪ Accessory/supernumerary nipple(s)
  - ▪ Axillary glandular tissue
  - ▪ Complete accessory breast in axilla

Management

- ▶ Annual screening mammography
- ▶ Further imaging or ultrasound only if concerning or symptomatic
  - ▪ Comparison with previous exams helpful
  - ▪ Spot views may be helpful on baseline exam to exclude underlying suspicious findings

Selected References/Further Reading

Adler DD, et al. Accessory breast tissue in the axilla: mammographic appearance. *Radiology* 1997;163:709-711.
Down S, et al. Management of accessory breast tissue in the axilla. *Br J Surg* 2003;90:1213-1214.

History

▶ Screening mammogram in a woman with a BRCA1 gene mutation. Additional clinical history withheld

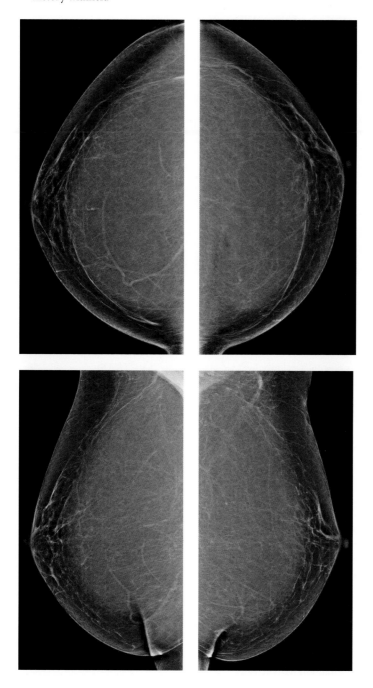

Case 86 Bilateral Transverse Rectus Abdominis Myocutaneous (TRAM) Flap Reconstructions

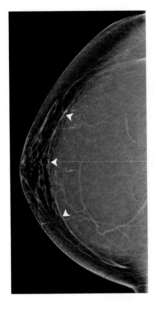 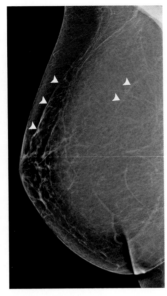

Findings

- ▶ Bilateral fatty tissue with complete absence of fibroglandular tissue
- ▶ Note the non-anatomic bands (*arrowheads*)
- ▶ The nipple-areolar complex (NAC) was reconstructed in this patient
- ▶ The patient is status post bilateral prophylactic mastectomies with TRAM reconstruction

Differential Diagnosis

- ▶ Other autologous tissue breast reconstructions such as deep inferior epigastric perforator (DIEP), latissimus dorsi myocutaneous (LDM), gluteal free flap, or lateral transverse thigh flap
- ▶ Reduction mammoplasty (absence of NAC and clinical history will differentiate)

Teaching Points

- ▶ Breast reconstruction is most often non-autologous
  - ▪ Tissue expanders and/or implants
- ▶ TRAM flap is the most common method of autologous breast reconstruction
  - ▪ Multiple techniques
    - ◆ Pedicle
    - ◆ Free flap
    - ◆ Delayed flap
  - ▪ Other tissue flaps can be used (as noted in the differential diagnosis)
- ▶ Classically, mammography depicts
  - ▪ Predominantly radiolucent (fatty) tissue
  - ▪ Muscular pedicle may be visible posteriorly on MLO views
  - ▪ Posterior surgical clips

- Non-anatomic bands
- No NAC
  - Although may have reconstructed NAC
    - Soft tissue and tattoo for pigmentation
► Fat necrosis common
- Most often seen in the periphery where blood supply is most tenuous
► Palpable mass in TRAM or soft tissue mass is much more likely to be fat necrosis than recurrence
- First-line imaging evaluation should be with mammography
  - Can demonstrate classic fat necrosis (which has a more variable appearance at ultrasound)
► MR may demonstrate a spectrum of findings
- Normal
- Expected postoperative changes including
  - Fibrosis, fat necrosis, skin thickening, seroma

Management

► Surveillance with clinical exam
► Routine mammographic screening of soft-tissue reconstructions is controversial and not routinely recommended by most breast imaging radiologists

Selected References/Further Reading

Bland K, Copeland E. *The Breast: Comprehensive Management of Benign and Malignant Disorders.* St. Louis, MO: Saunders, 2004: Chapter 43.

Devon RK, et al. Breast reconstruction with a transverse rectus abdominis myocutaneous flap: Spectrum of normal and abnormal MR Imaging findings. *RadioGraphics* 2004;24:1287-1299.

Hogge JP, et al. Mammography of autologous myocutaneous flaps. *RadioGraphics* 1999;19:S63-72.

History

▶ Abnormal screening mammogram. Left breast diagnostic mammogram images shown

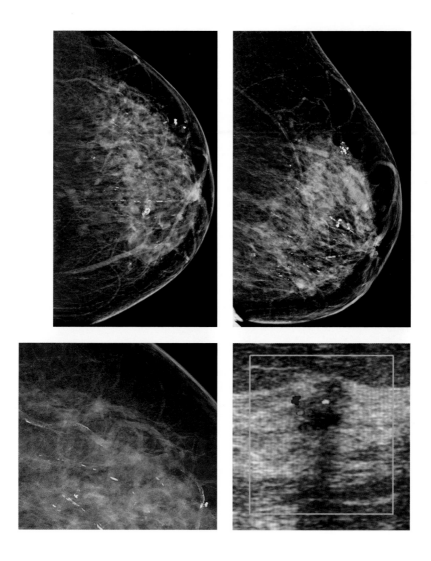

Case 87 Invasive Ductal Carcinoma (Low Grade)

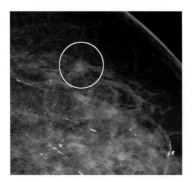

Findings

- ► Mammogram
  - Very small irregular mass with spiculated margins and associated architectural distortion, best seen on the full CC and spot magnification CC views (*circle*)
- ► Ultrasound
  - Small, irregular, hypoechoic mass with microlobulated margins and associated posterior acoustic shadowing

Differential Diagnosis

- ► Invasive lobular carcinoma
- ► Tubular carcinoma
- ► Radial scar

Teaching Points

- ► Finding very small early cancers in dense breast tissue requires high-quality imaging
- ► Radiologists can improve their ability to detect smaller lesions by
  - Comparing with prior exams when available
  - Learning and applying search patterns
  - Understanding subtle signs of malignancy
  - Working in a darkened room without distractions
  - Interpreting both screening and diagnostic exams
  - Resisting satisfaction of search when one abnormality is detected
- ► Reviewing false-negative exams as part of an annual audit may help improve performance

Management

- ► Ultrasound-guided core needle biopsy for tissue diagnosis
  - If ultrasound did not demonstrate a correlate for the mammographic findings, tissue sampling with stereotactic core needle biopsy is appropriate
- ► Consider breast MR for further evaluation once diagnosis of cancer confirmed
  - Extent of disease in the affected breast
  - Ancillary screening of the contralateral breast

Selected References/Further Reading

Majid ASD, et al. Missed breast carcinoma: pitfalls and pearls. *Radiographics* 2003;23:881-895.
Tabar L, et al. *Breast Cancer: The Art and Science of Early Detection with Mammography.* New York: Thieme, 2005.

History

► 34-year-old woman with a palpable breast mass and skin thickening, not improving with antibiotic therapy

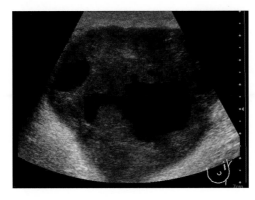 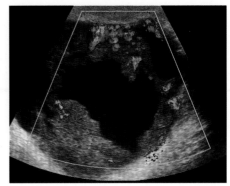

Left breast, upper outer quadrant

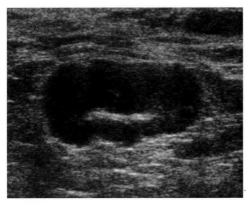

Axilla

Case 88 High-grade Invasive Ductal Carcinoma (Clinically Mistaken for an Abscess)

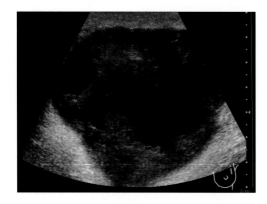
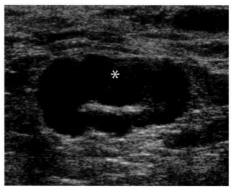

Findings

► Large heterogeneous complex mass with thick internal septations demonstrating increased vascularity on Doppler imaging
► Note the enlarged axillary lymph node with thickened cortex (asterisk)

Differential Diagnosis

► Abscess

Teaching Points

► Patients with clinical features suggesting breast infection should be followed carefully
  ▪ Failure to improve on appropriate antibiotic coverage is a worrisome sign
  ▪ Initially, inflammatory breast carcinoma may have similar clinical presentation to mastitis
► Large (greater than 2 cm) invasive carcinomas are prone to central necrosis
  ▪ Rapid growth results in decreased vascularity centrally as tumor outgrows blood supply
► Necrosis most common in high-grade invasive carcinoma NOS (not otherwise specified)

Management

► Ultrasound-guided core needle biopsy for tissue diagnosis
  ▪ Target the solid portion for best tissue sampling
  ▪ Fine-needle aspiration of the suspicious lymph node
► Bilateral mammography to evaluate extent of disease and screen the contralateral breast
► Once the diagnosis of malignancy is confirmed, contrast enhanced MR for additional evaluation (extent of disease and ancillary screening of the contralateral breast)

Selected References/Further Reading

Ikeda DM. *Breast Imaging: The Requisites*. Philadelphia: Elsevier Mosby, 2004:126-128.
Stavros AT. *Breast Ultrasound*. Philadelphia: Lippincott Williams & Wilkins, 2004:633-634.

History

▶ Patient with biopsy-proven left breast cancer undergoing neoadjuvant chemotherapy

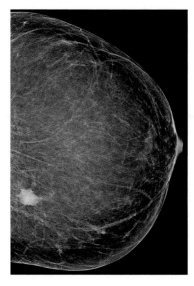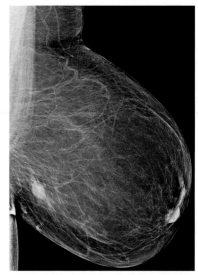

Baseline exam

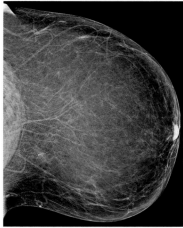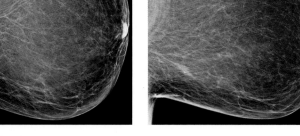

16 weeks after chemotherapy

Case 89   Favorable Response to Neoadjuvant Chemotherapy

Findings

▶ Baseline mammogram demonstrates a mass in the lower inner quadrant of the left breast (known biopsy-proven cancer)

▶ Repeat mammogram 16 weeks later demonstrates a tissue marker clip that was placed at the time of biopsy, no residual measurable mass, with minimal residual density

Teaching Points

▶ Currently, many patients with large tumors are given neo-adjuvant chemotherapy which consists of anti-cancer agents (may include endocrine therapy) to shrink mass(es) *prior* to definitive surgical treatment
  ▪ More common at tertiary care centers
  ▪ Performed both on and off clinical trial protocols

▶ Methods of assessing treatment response are available, but vary in applicability depending on individual patients, specific medications and imaging modalities used
  ▪ World Health Organization (WHO) set criteria for assessing treatment response in 1979
  ▪ Response Evaluation Criteria in Solid Tumors (RECIST) guidelines, established in 2000, clarify and further codify methods for assessing treatment response

▶ Terms applied to both clinical assessments of measuring and imaging measurement
  ▪ Complete response
  ▪ Partial response
  ▪ Stable disease
  ▪ Progressive disease

▶ For breast imaging, precise measurement in one, two, or three dimensions can be made using mammography, ultrasound, and MR
  ▪ Many digital imaging applications are capable of assessing area or volume of masses
    ◆ May be a more accurate assessment of response
    ◆ Not specifically used in most clinical trials
  ▪ Mammographic density often decreases with response to treatment, but this is even harder to quantify
  ▪ MR may be useful in assessing response, although, due to marked variability of effect on vascularity, may over- or under-estimate actual tumor size

▶ Tumor grade and extensive intraductal component (EIC) also affect the accuracy of preoperative measurements

Management

▶ Innumerable factors affect measurement accuracy across all imaging modalities
  ▪ Use measurements as a guide without dictating treatment decisions

▶ Best methods for obtaining and reporting imaging measurements will vary depending on the setting (investigational or clinical)

▶ Definitive surgery is performed when neo-adjuvant chemotherapy is completed

Selected References/Further Reading

Chagpar AB, et al. Accuracy of physical examination, ultrasonography, and mammography in predicting residual pathologic tumor size in patients treated with neoadjuvant chemotherapy. *Ann Surg* 2006;243:257-263.

Therasse P, et al. New guidelines to evaluate the response to treatment in solid tumors European Organization for Research and Treatment of Cancer, National Cancer Institute of the United States, National Cancer Institute of Canada. *J Natl Cancer Inst* 2000;92:205-216.

Wasser K, et al. Accuracy of tumor size measurement in breast cancer using MRI is influenced by histological regression induced by neoadjuvant chemotherapy. *Eur Radiol* 2003;13:1213-1223.

History

▶ Select non-contrast MR silicone-sensitive images from two patients (with the same diagnosis) are shown. Both patients have silicone breast implants

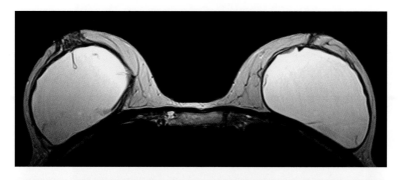

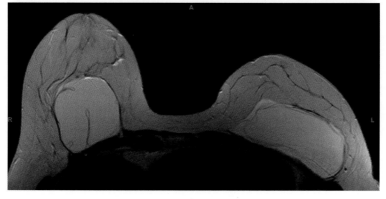

Case 90 Intracapsular Rupture of Silicone Implants (MR Appearance)

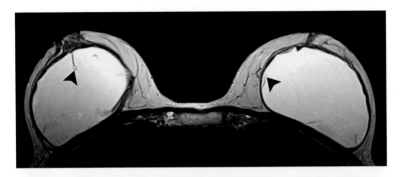

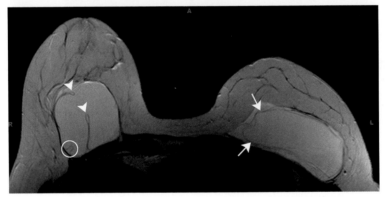

Findings

- Non-contrast MR: Silicone-sensitive sequence image demonstrates a "keyhole" sign (*black arrowheads*)
- Selected image from the second patient depicts the "linguine" sign (*white arrows*), the "noose" sign (*circle*), and "keyhole" signs (*white arrowheads*)

Differential Diagnosis

- Normal radial folds can mimic intracapsular rupture

Teaching Points

- Non-contrast MR is the modality of choice to detect intracapsular rupture
- Implants are not "lifetime devices"
- Use a dedicated breast coil
- Sequences may include
  - T2 weighted spin echo
  - Silicone-sensitive sequences
  - Axial and sagittal acquisitions
- Signs of intracapsular rupture
  - Linguine sign: dark lines within the implant indicating complete collapse of the implant envelope within the fibrous capsule
    - Most sensitive sign

- Keyhole sign: silicone present between the fibrous capsule and the uncollapsed envelope (also known as "inverted teardrop" or "noose")
- Water droplets: round areas that follow water signal intensity on all sequences
  - Low specificity
► Clinical history important to avoid false-positives
  - Know the type of implant
    - May misdiagnose double-lumen or stacked implants as ruptured
  - Silicone implants injected with saline or antibiotics during implantation
    - Water droplets may mimic microperforation
  - Extracapsular rupture from previous implants may confound imaging
    - Current implant may be entirely intact, despite the presence of "free" silicone
► Trace peri-implant fluid is commonly seen on T2-weighted images
  - Large collections may indicate infection
► FDA recommends non-contrast screening MR 3 years after placement of silicone implants and every 2 years thereafter to evaluate implant integrity
► Non-contrast breast MR is *not* intended to detect breast cancer
► MR should not be used in the evaluation of *saline* implants

Management

► Implant revision is performed based on patient wishes and the recommendations of her plastic surgeon

Selected References/Further Reading

Middleton MS, McNamara MP. *Breast Implant Imaging*. Philadelphia: Lippincott Williams & Wilkins, 2003.

Morris EA, Liberman L. *Breast MRI: Diagnosis and Intervention*. New York: Springer, 2005: Chapter 15.

Soo MS, et al. Intracapsular implant rupture: MR findings of incomplete shell collapse. *J Magn Reson Imaging* 1997;7:724-730.

History

▶ 40-year-old woman at high risk for developing breast cancer (Gail score = 28%). Contrast MR MIP (maximum intensity projection) image shown

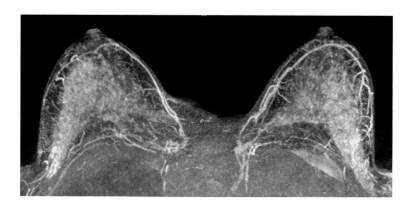

Case 91   Normal Background Glandular Enhancement

Findings

▶ MIP image demonstrates bilateral symmetric intense enhancement consistent with background enhancement (BE)
- This patient was imaged in the third week of her menstrual cycle

Differential Diagnosis

▶ Classic appearance demonstrated
▶ Fibrocystic change
▶ When focal or asymmetric, may mimic malignancy

Teaching Points

▶ Glandular tissue normally demonstrates enhancement
▶ Extensive ("marked" or "severe") BE may reduce sensitivity and specificity
- Can obscure abnormality and/or cause false-positives
▶ Does not necessarily correlate with mammographic density
▶ Varies during menstrual cycle (more pronounced in the first and fourth weeks)
- Ideal to image patients in the second week (days 7 to 14)
  ◆ Important for screening patients
  ◆ Do not delay imaging in patients with new cancer diagnosis
▶ Postmenopausal patients on HRT may have increased BE
▶ BE typically decreases in patients status post breast conserving surgery (lumpectomy and radiation therapy)
▶ Tamoxifen reduces background enhancement
▶ Indications for contrast enhanced breast MR
- Screening high-risk women in conjunction with annual mammography (American Cancer Society guidelines)
  ◆ BRCA mutation or first-degree relative with known BRCA mutation
  ◆ Calculated lifetime risk >20% to 25%
  ◆ Radiation to chest between ages 10 and 30
  ◆ Few rare genetic syndromes
- Diagnostic evaluation
  ◆ New diagnosis of cancer
    ◆ Evaluate extent of disease
      – Especially important in young patients, and those with tumors having lobular histology
    ◆ Screening the contralateral breast
    ◆ Evaluate for pectoralis muscle invasion
  ◆ Evaluating patients with metastatic axillary disease for possible occult breast malignancy
  ◆ Response to neoadjuvant chemotherapy
  ◆ Not typically used for problem solving
    ◆ Not for pain, lump, or other clinical problem that should be evaluated with mammography/ultrasound
    ◆ Should not dissuade biopsy of a finding that is suspicious on mammography or ultrasound

- ▶ Considerations/recommendations for contrast MR technique and reporting
  - ▪ Have recent mammogram for correlation
  - ▪ Check renal function as warranted
  - ▪ Use a dedicated breast coil
  - ▪ Obtain bilateral imaging
  - ▪ Use BI-RADS® lexicon terminology in reports
    - ◆ Describe morphology and kinetics
  - ▪ Include succinct management recommendations
- ▶ ACR accreditation for breast MR now available

Management

- ▶ Annual screening mammography and annual screening MR, given high-risk status

Selected References/Further Reading

Lehman CD, et al. Screening women at high risk for breast cancer with mammography and magnetic resonance imaging. *Cancer* 2005;103:1898-1905.

Morris EA, Liberman L. *Breast MRI: Diagnosis and Intervention*. New York: Springer, 2005.

Saslow D, et al. American Cancer Society guidelines for breast screening with MRI as an adjunct to mammography. *CA: Cancer J Clinicians* 2007;57:75-89.

History

▶ 55-year-old woman with newly diagnosed breast cancer

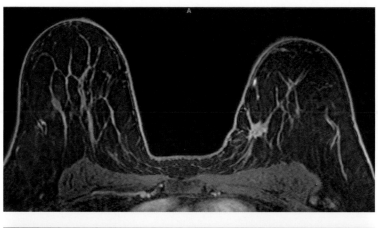

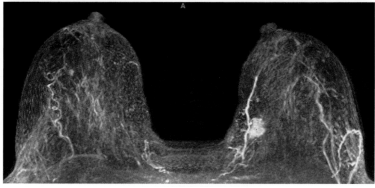

Case 92 Invasive Ductal Carcinoma

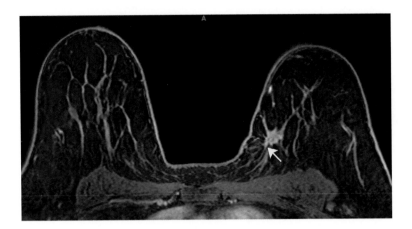

Findings

▶ Contrast enhanced images depicts an irregular enhancing mass with spiculated margins (*arrow*) demonstrating mixed contrast kinetics including washout component
  ▪ Note the slight skin retraction superficial to the tumor

Differential Diagnosis

▶ Invasive lobular carcinoma

Teaching Points

▶ MR does not replace thorough mammographic and sonographic evaluation of patients with suspicious clinical or imaging findings
▶ Tumor angiogenesis is postulated to explain lesion enhancement
▶ Morphology is the most important feature to consider in evaluating lesions on MR
  ▪ Contrast kinetic information is more critical to determining the possibility of malignancy in cases with more benign-appearing morphology
▶ Classic appearance on MR depicts irregular, enhancing mass (+/- rim enhancement) with washout kinetic curve
  ▪ May have internal enhancing septations
  ▪ With the appearance in this case, the probability of malignancy approaches 100%
▶ Patients with a new cancer diagnosis may benefit from breast MR, especially those with dense parenchyma on mammography
  ▪ MR evaluates extent of disease in the affected breast and serves for ancillary screening of the contralateral breast

Management

▶ Breast conserving therapy (lumpectomy and radiation therapy)

Selected References/Further Reading

Liberman L. MR imaging of the ipsilateral breast in women with percutaneously proven breast cancer. *AJR* 2003;180:901-910.

Morris EA, Liberman L. *Breast MRI: Diagnosis and Intervention*. New York: Springer, 2005: 51-78 and 79-80.

History

▶ 42-year-old woman at high risk for developing breast cancer (Gail score = 38%). MIP (maximum intensity projection) image from baseline screening breast MR shown

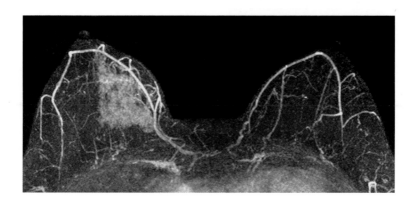

Case 93   Ductal Carcinoma In Situ (DCIS)

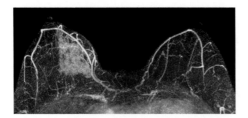

Findings

▶ Contrast enhanced MR demonstrates abnormal segmental enhancement in the right medial breast. Kinetic analysis (not shown) demonstrated predominantly a plateau-curve enhancement pattern

Differential Diagnosis

▶ Fibrocystic change
▶ Asymmetric background enhancement

Teaching Points

▶ MR is extremely sensitive for the detection of breast malignancy
  ▪ Slightly diminished sensitivity for detection of DCIS
    ◆ Reported between 77% and 96%
▶ Classic MR appearance of DCIS depicts non-mass-like, clumped enhancement in linear or segmental distribution
  ▪ Variable kinetic curves reported
    ◆ Unreliable discriminator—persistent kinetic curve should not dissuade biopsy of a morphologically suspicious finding
▶ MR may depict true extent of non-calcified DCIS
  ▪ Consider MR in select patients with new diagnosis of DCIS
    ◆ Young
    ◆ Dense breasts mammographically
    ◆ Extensive calcifications with possible underlying invasive component

Management

▶ Tissue sampling is warranted for diagnosis, given the highly suspicious appearance of the right breast
  ▪ Correlation with current mammogram (evaluate for suspicious microcalcifications in the same distribution) that would permit targeting for stereotactic core needle biopsy
  ▪ If mammogram is normal, consider second-look ultrasound
    ◆ Lower yield for DCIS than a mass
  ▪ If ultrasound is normal, MR-guided biopsy is recommended for tissue diagnosis

Selected References/Further Reading

Jansen SA, et al. Pure ductal carcinoma in situ: kinetic and morphologic MR characteristics compared with mammographic appearance and nuclear grade. *Radiology* 2007;245:684-691.
Menell JH, et al. Determination of the presence and extent of pure ductal carcinoma in situ by mammography and magnetic resonance imaging. *Breast J* 2005;11:382-390.
Orel SG, et al. MR imaging of ductal carcinoma in situ. *Radiology* 1997;202:413-420.

History

▶ 39-year-old woman at high risk for developing breast cancer (Gail score = 21%). MIP (maximum intensity projection) image from baseline screening breast MR shown

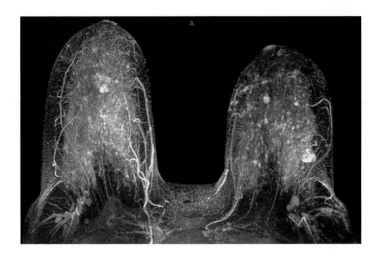

Case 94 Bilateral Fibroadenomas (FA)

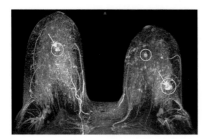

Findings

▶ Contrast enhanced MR demonstrates bilateral multiple enhancing masses (*circles*) with similar imaging features: circumscribed, oval, homogeneously enhancing with non-enhancing internal septations (*arrows*). Kinetic analyses (not shown) demonstrate persistent enhancement curves

Differential Diagnosis

▶ Classic appearance demonstrated (multiplicity and imaging findings)
▶ If isolated to one mass, consider more suspicious etiology (malignancy)
   ▪ *Caveat:* In high-risk patients, especially those with BRCA mutations, malignancy can masquerade as benign findings

Teaching Points

▶ Most common benign solid breast mass
▶ Classic MR appearance depicts oval, circumscribed, +/- gentle lobulation, homogeneously enhancing mass with or without non-enhancing internal septations
   ▪ Non-enhancing internal septations
      ◆ High negative predictive value: very specific sign of FA
         ◦ Not always present
   ▪ Kinetic analysis is variable but classically demonstrates persistent enhancement
   ▪ May have increased T2 signal, but variable
      ◆ Nonspecific discriminator
   ▪ Degenerating FA may not enhance
▶ Rarely phyllodes tumor can masquerade as FA on MR

Management

▶ Correlation with recent mammogram may demonstrate bilateral degenerating fibroadenomas (masses with coarse or "popcorn" calcifications)
▶ Given the multiplicity and classic appearance of non-enhancing internal septations, annual mammography and MR were recommended. The above findings have been stable for more than 3 years
▶ If atypical features (morphology or kinetic curve) are present, or solitary finding, second-look ultrasound should be performed for additional evaluation
   ▪ If new or enlarging, tissue diagnosis is warranted

Selected References/Further Reading

Hochman MG, et al. Fibroadenoma: MR imaging appearances with radiologic-histopathologic correlations. *Radiology* 1997;204:123-129.
Morris EA, Liberman L. *Breast MRI: Diagnosis and Intervention*. New York: Springer, 2005:115-123.

History

► 58-year-old woman status post left breast excisional biopsy at an outside facility. Biopsy yielded invasive ductal carcinoma with multiple positive margins. MR was requested for surgical planning. Select post-contrast images and color overlay MIP images shown (color to depict kinetics)

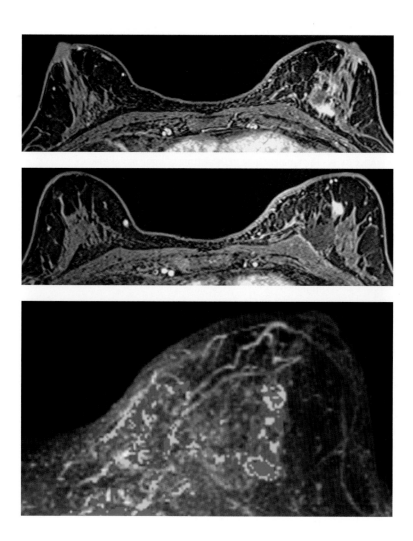

Case 95 Residual Invasive Ductal Carcinoma

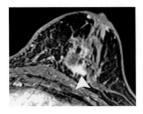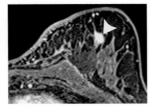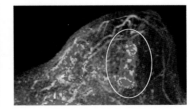

Findings

▶ Contrast MR demonstrates homogeneously low signal in the biopsy cavity (corresponding high T2 signal, not shown) with multiple adjacent irregular, enhancing masses (*arrowheads*) demonstrating predominantly "washout" kinetics (red indicates washout on color MIP, *circle*)

Differential Diagnosis

▶ Classic appearance for residual malignancy in the setting of known malignancy and positive surgical margins

Teaching Points

▶ MR is helpful to assess for residual disease in patients with close or positive margins at the time of surgical excision, especially in cases with:
  ▪ Dense breasts mammographically
  ▪ Tumors with invasive lobular histology
  ▪ Extensive intraductal component (EIC)
▶ May be more reliable if performed 3 to 4 weeks postoperatively
▶ Thick, nodular, or irregular enhancement at biopsy site is highly suspicious
▶ Thin (<5 mm) enhancing rim around biopsy cavity is expected, but in the setting of positive margins, re-excision is still warranted
  ▪ Microscopic disease not reliably imaged
▶ If suspicious calcifications are present on the preoperative mammogram, a post-excision mammogram is helpful to assess for residual suspicious calcifications
  ▪ Suspicious calcifications are highly predictive for residual disease
  ▪ Mammography is more limited to assess for residual masses and/or architectural distortion due to expected postoperative changes

Management

▶ Re-excision in attempt to achieve acceptable negative margins
  ▪ Surgeon can be alerted to areas of bulky residual disease
    ◆ Assist in surgical planning
  ▪ If distant lesion is detected that might preclude breast conserving surgery, second-look ultrasound and biopsy would be warranted

Selected References/Further Reading

Frei KA, et al. MR imaging of the breast in patients with positive margins after lumpectomy: influence of the time interval between lumpectomy and MR imaging. *AJR* 2000;175:1577-1584.
Lee CH. Problem solving MR imaging of the breast. *Radiol Clin North Am* 2004;42:919-934.
Morris EA, Liberman L. *Breast MRI: Diagnosis and Intervention.* New York: Springer, 2005: Chapter 13.

History

▶ 48 year-old woman with known cancer in the right upper outer quadrant in a patient with extremely dense breasts. Select images from contrast-enhanced breast MR shown

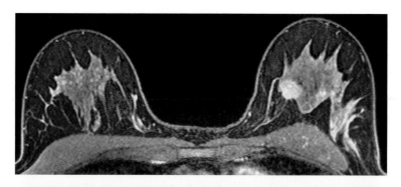

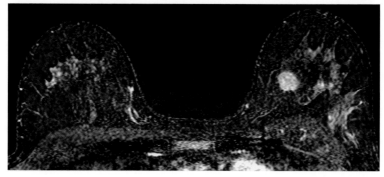

Case 96   Contralateral Synchronous Cancer Detected by MR

Findings

▶ MR demonstrates a heterogeneously enhancing mass with lobular margins in the left inner breast. Contrast kinetics analysis showed a dominant washout curve
  ▪ Known cancer in the right breast was also visible (not shown) and had similar imaging features

Differential Diagnosis

▶ Invasive lobular cancer
▶ Benign solid mass unlikely, given the highly suspicious features

Teaching Points

▶ MR detects contralateral breast cancer in 3% to 8% of patients
▶ Synchronous bilateral cancer
  ▪ Within 3 to 12 months following diagnosis of index cancer (exact timeframe variably defined)
  ▪ Prevalence of synchronous bilateral breast cancer is 1% to 3%
  ▪ Higher risk for multicentric disease
▶ Metachronous contralateral cancer
  ▪ Subsequent contralateral cancer (>12 months following diagnosis of index cancer)
  ▪ Risk estimate is approximately1% per year following diagnosis of index cancer
▶ MR should be considered in patients with new diagnosis of breast cancer, especially those with
  ▪ Young age
  ▪ Mammographically dense breasts
  ▪ Lobular tumor histology
  ▪ Family history
▶ MR has high sensitivity which may lead to false-positive findings
  ▪ Patients should be counseled about the potential for additional imaging (second-look ultrasound) and procedures (additional biopsies)

Management

▶ Second-look ultrasound in order to perform ultrasound-guided core needle biopsy
  ▪ If mass could not be detected with ultrasound, then MR biopsy for diagnosis would be required
▶ Patients presenting with bilateral cancer have a higher risk for genetic mutation
  ▪ Consider genetic counseling

Selected References/Further Reading

Lee SG, et al. MR imaging screening of the contralateral breast in patients with newly diagnosed breast cancer: preliminary results. *Radiology* 2003;226: 773-778.

Lehman CD, et al. Indications for breast MRI in the patient with newly diagnosed breast cancer. *J Natl Compr Canc Network JNCCN* 2009;7:193-201.

Morris EA, Liberman L. *Breast MRI: Diagnosis and Intervention.* New York: Springer, 2005, 207-211.

History

▶ 44-year-old woman with newly diagnosed breast cancer

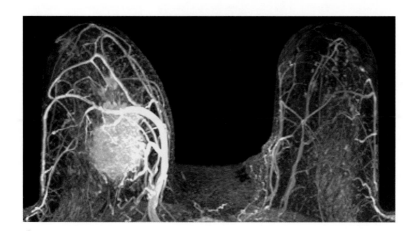

Case 97   Invasive Lobular Carcinoma (ILC)

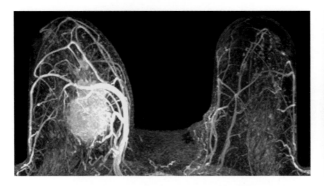
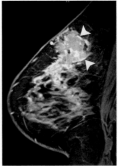

Findings

▶ MIP image depicts a large enhancing irregular mass in the upper inner right breast. Sagittal post-contrast image demonstrates an irregular mass with rim enhancement (*arrowheads*). Note the enlarged vessels in the right breast

Differential Diagnosis

▶ Invasive ductal carcinoma (IDC)

Teaching Points

▶ Second most common breast carcinoma
  ▪ 10% to 15% of all invasive breast cancers
▶ Higher rate of multiplicity and bilaterality compared to IDC
▶ MR is more sensitive than mammography and ultrasound in assessing
  ▪ Multifocal and/or multicentric tumors
  ▪ Tumor size (classically underestimated with mammography and ultrasound)
▶ MR is helpful for preoperative surgical planning
  ▪ Mastectomy may be required when more extensive disease is documented
    ◆ If patient is motivated for breast conserving surgery, additional biopsies should be performed to document true extent
▶ Variable MR appearance but classically depicts solitary, irregular enhancing mass with spiculated margins, +/- rim enhancement
  ▪ May have diffuse enhancement pattern mimicking normal glandular tissue
  ▪ Enhancing strands may be seen amidst multiple enhancing foci
  ▪ Contrast kinetics are variable, but majority have delayed enhancement resulting in plateau or persistent contrast enhancement curves
    ◆ May increase false-negative exams if not recognized

Management

▶ Breast conservation therapy (lumpectomy and radiation therapy) or mastectomy, depending on extent

Selected References/Further Reading

Lopez JK, Bassett LW. Invasive lobular carcinoma of the breast: spectrum of mammographic, US and MR imaging findings. *RadioGraphics* 2009;29:165-176.

Morris EA, Liberman L. *Breast MRI: Diagnosis and Intervention.* New York: Springer, 2005:209.

History

▶ 52-year-old woman with a newly diagnosed left breast cancer

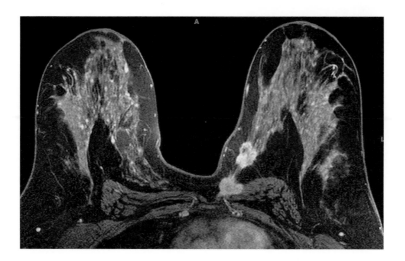

Case 98   Breast Cancer with Invasion of the Pectoralis Muscle

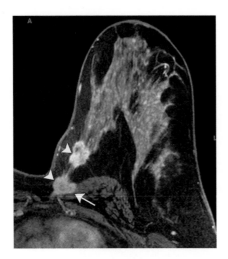

Findings

▶ Contrast MR demonstrates two heterogeneously enhancing spiculated masses in the left upper inner quadrant (*arrowheads*). The posterior mass directly invades the pectoralis muscle (*arrow*)

Differential Diagnosis

▶ Classic appearance demonstrated

Teaching Points

▶ Accurate evaluation of deep/posterior tumors is critical for treatment planning and staging; however, assessing pectoralis muscle involvement with clinical exam and imaging can be difficult
  ▪ MR is an excellent modality to assess for possible pectoralis muscle invasion
▶ Involvement of the pectoralis fascia/muscle or chest wall may prompt neoadjuvant chemotherapy or more aggressive surgery
  ▪ A portion of the fascia/muscle may require excision
▶ Pectoralis muscle normally enhances following contrast administration
▶ Tumor involvement shows infiltrative enhancement or mass-like enhancement
  ▪ Abnormal enhancement highly predictive of true invasion
  ▪ True invasion is unlikely when a mass directly abuts the muscle (obliteration of the intervening fat plane) but normal pectoralis enhancement is observed

Management

▶ Document extent of disease in order to direct treatment planning
▶ Consider follow-up imaging during and after neoadjuvant chemotherapy to assess response

Selected References/Further Reading

Morris EA, et al. Evaluation of the pectoralis major muscle in patients with posterior breast tumors on breast MR images: early experience. *Radiology* 2000;214:67-72.
Morris EA, Liberman L. *Breast MRI: Diagnosis and Intervention.* New York: Springer, 2005:34.

History

▶ 35-year-old woman with newly diagnosed 2.2-cm right breast cancer (high grade invasive ductal carcinoma). The patient has extremely dense breasts mammographically

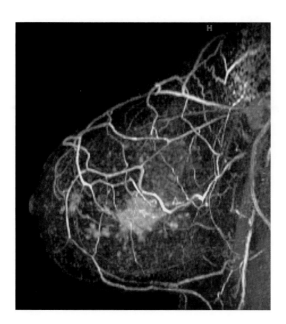

Case 99 Multifocal Carcinoma (True Disease Extent Demonstrated on MR Imaging)

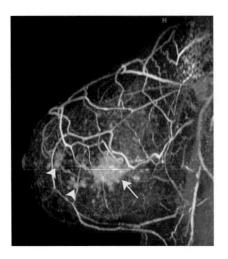

Findings

► Sagittal MIP image from contrast MR demonstrates the known index tumor: a lobulated heterogeneously enhancing mass (*arrow*)
► Multiple additional, smaller, enhancing masses are present in a segmental distribution (*arrowheads* indicate two representative lesions)
► All masses demonstrated similar washout contrast kinetics (not shown)

Differential Diagnosis

► Papillomatosis/Multiple papillomas
► Benign masses or fibrocystic change (highly unlikely given the appearance and distribution)

Teaching Points

► Multifocal breast cancer is associated with higher local recurrence rates
  ▪ May preclude breast conservation therapy
    ♦ Consider extent versus breast size to achieve acceptable surgical margins and aesthetic outcome
► Wide variation (6% to 34%) reported in MR sensitivity for detecting additional ipsilateral disease
► MR is especially helpful to determine ipsilateral extent of disease in women with
  ▪ Young age
  ▪ Mammographically dense breasts
  ▪ Lobular tumor histology
  ▪ BRCA mutation
► MR has a high positive predictive value when there is a suspicious finding in the same breast as the known cancer
► MR has lower specificity than sensitivity
  ▪ Biopsy should be performed to confirm diagnosis, given the possibility for false positive findings

- Surgical decision making should be based on biopsy-proven findings rather than imaging appearance alone in patients motivated for breast conserving therapy (BCT)
  - Not all "suspicious" findings on MR are malignant

Management

- Directed, second-look ultrasound of MR findings, to perform ultrasound-guided core needle biopsy and document true extent of disease
  - If the MR findings cannot be reliably detected with ultrasound, then MR biopsy for definitive diagnosis may be required

Selected References/Further Reading

Liberman L, et al. MR Imaging of the ipsilateral breast in women with percutaneously proven breast cancer. *AJR* 2003;180:901-910.

Meissnitzer M, et al. Targeted ultrasound of the breast in women with abnormal MRI findings for whom biopsy has been recommended. *AJR* 2009;193:1025-1029.

Morris EA, Liberman L. *Breast MRI: Diagnosis and Intervention.* New York: Springer, 2005: Chapter 23.

History

▶ 46-year-old woman with an abnormal screening mammogram. Screening images and spot magnification view are shown. Ultrasound failed to demonstrate a correlate for the mammographic finding. Past surgical history includes explantation of silicone implants

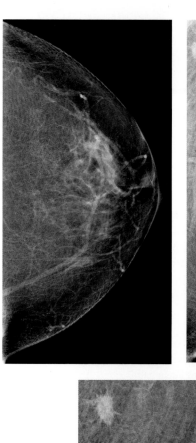
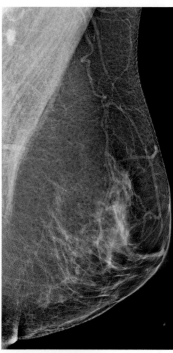
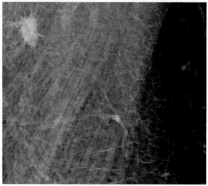

Case 100 Silicone-Laden Lymph Node Mimicking Cancer on a Mammogram

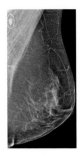 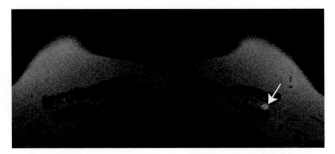

Findings

▶ Mammogram: Spiculated focal asymmetry with "mass-like" features (convex borders) in the deep upper breast on the MLO view (*circle*). No correlate is present on the CC view

▶ Given the lack of ultrasound correlate for the mammographic finding, and the history of prior silicone implants, a non-contrast breast MR was performed to pursue the possibility of silicone granuloma/silicone adenopathy

  ▪ A silicone-sensitive sequence confirms silicone in a sub-pectoral lymph node (*arrow*). This accounts for the mammographic finding (and the anatomic location explains the inability to visualize on ultrasound imaging)

Differential Diagnosis

▶ With only the mammogram finding

  ▪ Invasive ductal carcinoma
  ▪ Invasive lobular carcinoma
  ▪ Occult breast primary malignancy with metastatic adenopathy

▶ With addition of the MR, classic finding of silicone adenopathy demonstrated

Teaching Points

▶ Clinical correlation can be critical to image interpretation, including

  ▪ Past surgical history
    ◆ Benign
    ◆ Malignant
    ◆ Cosmetic
  ▪ Known diagnoses
    ◆ Systemic illness (e.g., collagen vascular disease)
    ◆ Genetic disorders (e.g., neurofibromatosis)

▶ MR should not typically used for "problem solving" but was critical in this case

  ▪ Meticulous diagnostic mammography, in conjunction with ultrasound, overwhelmingly resolves questionable mammographic findings
  ▪ MR should *never* be first-line imaging for screen-detected findings

- ▸ Rarely, MR may be indicated when mammography is problematic (after thorough diagnostic evaluation is completed)
  - ▪ Questionable architectural distortion
  - ▪ Questionable new focal asymmetry
  - ▪ One-view suspicious finding
    - ◆ Assists in lesion localization and permits accurate second-look ultrasound
  - ▪ Scar versus recurrent tumor

Management

- ▸ Patient reassurance and annual screening mammography

Selected References/Further Reading

Lee CH. Problem solving MR imaging of the breast. *Radiol Clin North Am* 2004;42:919-934.
Morris EA, Liberman L. *Breast MRI: Diagnosis and Intervention.* New York: Springer, 2005: Chapter 15.

Index of Cases

Index

Index